EMBRYO CULTURE

SARAH CRICHTON BOOKS
FARRAR, STRAUS AND GIROUX
NEW YORK

EMBRYO CULTURE

Making Babies

in the

Twenty-first

Century

BETH KOHL

Sarah Crichton Books
Farrar, Straus and Giroux
19 Union Square West, New York 10003

Distributed in Canada by Douglas & McIntyre Ltd.
Printed in the United States of America
First edition, 2007

Library of Congress Cataloging-in-Publication Data
Kohl, Beth, 1968–
    Embryo culture : making babies in the twenty-first century / Beth
Kohl.—1st ed.
        p. cm.
    "Sarah Crichton Books."
    ISBN-13: 978-0-374-14757-0 (hardcover : alk. paper)
    ISBN-10: 0-374-14757-4 (hardcover : alk. paper)
    1. Kohl, Beth, 1968– —Health.   2. Infertility—Patients—Biography.
3. Fertilization in vitro, Human—Popular works.   I. Title.

RG135.K64   2007
618.1'780092—dc22
[B]
                                                        2007000893

Designed by Debbie Glasserman

www.fsgbooks.com

1   3   5   7   9   10   8   6   4   2

FOR GARY, SOPHIA, ANNA, AND LILY

AUTHOR'S NOTE

Many of the names and identifying characteristics of people and institutions I encountered have been changed, and much of the dialogue has inevitably been reconstructed. Websites may have changed or disappeared between when this book was written and when it is read. Further, the fact that an organization or website is referred to as a citation and/or a potential source of further information does not mean that the author or the publisher endorses the information the organization or website may provide or recommendations it may make.

CONTENTS

EMBRYO CULTURE

Materia Medica

Dr. Kevin Hamlin, Cape Town transplant, tan and animated, rolls to a stop between my legs. Above the draped horizon appears a green paper cap, secured with four strings behind his head. I'm on an operating table onto which, moments earlier, a nurse had helped me, first supporting my elbow, then manually guiding my stocking feet into dual metal cups projecting from the table's edge. I've worn my lucky socks, the same ones I slept in the night before my wedding, the ones I wear when I fly.

The nurse is a motherly lady I've not seen before. Pre-op prep is her main job here, I learn, this in keeping with the Henry Ford principle of specialization essential to the high success rates of Great Lakes Fertility. She runs down some facts about the impending procedure, pausing between items to concentrate on arranging the room just so.

"Once we get going, it's real fast," she said, "two, three minutes tops." I found this reassuring, proof that I wasn't a test case and that they had the science down to a science. She positioned next to the table a tall wheeled cart upon which gleamed assorted metal instruments. Sharp skinny ones and more spoony-looking ones. From a drawer on the back side of the cart, she pulled out plastic-wrapped this and that.

"We've employed assisted hatching," she continued, "by placing a slit in the natural envelope surrounding the embryos. This increases the chances they'll implant in the lining of your uterus." She reached up, repositioned the overhead lights, squeezed my forearm reassuringly, and told me not to go anywhere, she'd be right back.

The room is filled with medical personnel: an ultrasonographer named George, a couple of men in scrubs who walk between the OR and the lab (which is just on the other side of an interior door), and Carol, the statuesque head nurse, her back to me while she fills out paperwork on a counter near the sink. The prep nurse darts in and out, rushing a bit and asking me repeatedly if I'm doing okay, still hanging in there. She tells Dr. Hamlin he's needed in the hall. She has left the door open, and I can see a man in scrubs, arms crossed as he leans against the wall. He smiles at me. (The business end of the table is angled away from the door, affording him a restricted view of my right profile.) I smile back.

"Sorry, Liz," Dr. Hamlin says, calling me what he normally calls me and not Beth, the name I've offered. "Be back in a flash. Not to worry."

I watch Dr. Hamlin. He slides off his hat and bunches it in his fist. Putting his arm around the man's shoulder, he leans in. The men talk softly, but I can hear Dr. Hamlin repeating "Yes, yes" and wonder whether this conversation concerns me. It must, I figure; otherwise why would Dr. Hamlin, who had already scrubbed in, be summoned at the precise moment we've all been working toward?

Perhaps the discussion concerns our embryos: they are missing. Rather, they are mutant, the cellular equivalent of an original animal model of unusual interest with respect to its phenotype. Maybe our embryonic cells are dividing at breakneck speed, growing so large and complex that they've started to resemble human infants, overflowing the edges of the petri dish even as they float in their culture. All they need to satisfy our quest for an adorable child is floaty wings and a schmear of zinc oxide on their embryonic noses. Or perhaps they are the wrong color, or starting to take on an ominous shape, little pentacles or scythes when viewed through the microscope. Our mutating embryos have forced these scientists and technicians to reconsider their absolute faith that life, at this very early stage, is nothing more than perfectly knowable amino acids and lipids.

It's probably office doings, I tell myself, nothing more than a worker asking the boss his opinion on an emergent situation. Somebody else's emergent situation. After all, here at Great Lakes Fertility, where the medications have been tweaked to the milliliter, where each patient is a distinct assemblage of issues and challenges, each embryo containing a unique chemistry and DNA profile, where the mission is to create actual people out of cells, actual parents out of people, there are bound to be a host of profoundly important matters at any given moment.

Still, it is hard for me to sit tight and watch Dr. Hamlin powwowing in the hall when his rightful place is back here before me, expertly wielding one end of a catheter whose terminus hovers within my uterus. And since I've become attuned over the past couple of months to watching for physical cues—specks of blood in the syringe with which I inject myself, cramps indicating hyperstimulation or a twisted ovary, tender breasts that could mean pregnancy or cancer—it is only natural that I'd endeavor to read these guys for hints.

Trying hard to remain calm, I decide to put this unforeseen break to productive use and think religious thoughts. I've recently been to synagogue, for the High Holy Days, and stumbled upon back-to-back passages that evoked not hosannas but misgivings over the connection between in vitro fertilization (IVF) and God. The first passage was a thank-you to God for our bodies, acknowledging His wisdom and precision, His adroit arrangement of veins and arteries and vital organs for a finely balanced system. He is referred to as a fashioner of life, and I'm hoping He, like Hamlin, is also wearing his fashioning hat this morning in case it is He, not Hamlin, who is responsible for how things will turn out.

The second benediction thanks God for bestowing our pure souls and for tending to the souls of the living and the spirits of all flesh. I wonder, if Dr. Hamlin succeeds in impregnating me, if the resulting child will lack a soul, having bypassed traditional modes of creation and all. I worry they'll be mere body parts, a void existing where God-given spirit should reside, my child doomed not only to no afterlife, if afterlife there is, but to an empty and limited earthly existence. How I wish I knew a special prayer for fertility, one for good luck and another promising God I'll be more observant and do more of His bidding if only He'll help me out at this important juncture. I kick myself for not having done my spiritual research.

I shift gears, trying to engage a visualization technique from my yoga class. Shutting my eyes, I conjure Dr. Hamlin. He's holding a syringe containing *materia medica* belonging to my husband, Gary, and me, a glimmering liquid in which are suspended the three best embryos as determined by Debbie, Dr. Hamlin's much-ballyhooed embryologist. The genetic potential we've worked so hard for, suffered indignities over, fought about, and avoided discussing with friends and family is a cool blue color, luminous as a lit swimming pool at night. Dr. Hamlin smiles and walks slowly toward me. Next I envision a teeny floating embryo, weightless and slow-moving as fish food. It travels gently yet purposefully toward the primed wall of my uterus, a quiet dark nook, the perfect spot in which to burrow and flourish.

Inhaling deeply, visualizing my lungs expanding, and gradually deflating to my backward count of ten, I open my eyes. Hamlin is coming back, and Gary, having finally found the right-size scrubs, follows behind. They walk toward me. Gary smiles gently as he takes up his post behind me. Hamlin replaces his hat, quickly looping its strings the same unconscious, mechanical way fingers have tied bows since man first lashed together the roofs of huts, adorned the braids of daughters, affixed digit reminders pre-Post-it. His hands are neat and strong, a surgeon's tidy, dexterous tools. The pre-op nurse helps him into a fresh pair of surgical gloves.

"Just a couple more secs," he says, patting my leg and jiggling the loose part of my inner thigh. "The folks in the lab like to make sure, and make sure again, that the embryos they deliver are rightfully yours."

At a loss for words, I smile, beseech my thigh to stop rocking, and hope that the much-anticipated embryos materialize not only soon but, eventually, into a baby. The spot on my thigh that Dr. Hamlin touched feels warmer than the rest of my leg. I envision the nimble way he tied his hat and pray the work he's about to do comes as naturally and automatically. After all, these procedures are hardly ancient medicine: 1978 marked the first in vitro success in England with the birth of Louise Brown, the name I remember from my own childhood as belonging to this alien life-form, a test tube baby. In 1981 the first successful IVF was performed in the United States, resulting in the birth of baby Elizabeth Carr. Today there are around 460 IVF clinics in the United States. The best report success rates of more than 30 percent per cycle after embryo transfer, even better than the 20 to 25 percent chance of natural pregnancy in any given month under ideal natural conditions. And Ms. Brown is in good company. In the United States in 2001 there were 40,000 babies born as a result of IVF. In 2002 close to 47,000 babies were born as a result of combined assisted-reproductive technologies (ART). In 2004 more than a million

Americans availed themselves of infertility services. And as of 2005 more than a million children have been born worldwide thanks to IVF.

Specialists have had plenty of time and patients on which to practice their craft and refine and perfect its methods. But with ever newer and better ways to guarantee the desired result of a healthy live birth and with constantly refined protocols for reducing the number of high-order multiples, I can imagine even the most highly skilled doctor leading a patient down the wrong path. Even with a relatively young patient, younger than thirty-five and certainly no older than her late forties, the drop-dead age for most certified clinics, I can imagine a scenario in which a doctor, concerned with his success rates and American Society for Reproductive Medicine (ASRM) accreditation, overdoes it.

He might transfer a reckless number of embryos back into the uterus, a Hail Mary attempt to get one to stick. So let's say it works, she gets pregnant. Then what? The doctor can add one more pregnancy to the tote board, even if it never results in a live birth (a different statistic and one that oftentimes is mentioned as an afterthought, like pregnancy's anticlimax). The woman is then forced to decide whether she could or would carry multiples to term, the danger being that the more fetuses, the greater the risk of complications, the greater the chance for miscarriage. Conversely, she must decide whether she could or would "selectively reduce" those much-wished-for, even if additional, pregnancies.

I've seen Dr. Hamlin's success rates, among the best in North America, and his S-Class Mercedes parked in the clinic lot. Hey, everyone has to make a living, and I consider this a wonderful way. This Mercedes-driving, Alps-skiing doc helps realize dreams (unlike, say, an anesthesiologist, who numbs people), allowing folks to confront their anxieties, pursue their biological imperatives, and fulfill their desires. He gives otherwise barren individuals a chance at procreating. And he does it without judging them or discriminating among them, except to level with those who, by virtue of an insurmountable medical obstacle, have to consider other, nonmedical options.

Dr. Hamlin is a kind of miracle worker, and I am glad his job is lucrative: happy doctor, happy patient. I just hope he doesn't rest on his laurels. I need him to be as ambitious as ever in my case, even if mine is the umpteenth uterus he's probed this month. I want to remind him that even though hundreds of thousands of American babies (and counting) have been born as a result of this technique, what was that compared with the billions of people conceived the regular way? A drop in the human bucket.

There are 6.1 million clinically infertile men and women in this country, according to the ASRM. Clinical infertility is defined as twelve months of unprotected intercourse without achieving pregnancy. Primary infertility, my diagnosis, is infertility without any previous pregnancy. Secondary infertility is when a previous pregnancy has been achieved. Sterility is when pregnancy is impossible. Infertility, unlike sterility, generally represents only a reduced potential for pregnancy.

Every year approximately 5 percent of the 6.1 million infertile Americans, or 300,000 women, take a clinical shot at reproducing via IVF. Typically IVF cycles begin by shutting down the ovaries with a medication known as a GnRH agonist, Lupron being the most common. After two weeks of this med, the ovaries are stimulated with a potent ovulation medication such as Pergonal, which is injected for around ten days. When the eggs are nearly ready for harvesting, hCG is injected to induce final maturation. The eggs are then harvested, a process called aspiration, which involves passing a thin needle through the vagina and into the ovaries under ultrasound guidance, to suction the eggs from the follicles. An average of five to fifteen eggs are collected and then fertilized either by introducing

around 100,000 motile sperm to each egg or by intracytoplasmic sperm injection (ICSI), which involves puncturing the
egg and injecting exactly one choice sperm.

For a person who places great faith in statistics and Western
medical advances, IVF, as tough a procedure as it is, is a pretty
good bet. During any given IVF cycle, including those undergone by younger and older women alike, those with two well-
functioning ovaries and others with a barely operational one,
the probability of a successful pregnancy is approximately
18 percent, with a "take-home baby rate" of around 14 percent.
And as dramatic as I consider my own experience with ART,
involving as it does creation, religious controversy, sexuality,
social and medical implications, and politics, I find comfort
in enacting the same drama as approximately 300,000 other
women. I find comfort, too, in knowing that Louise Brown, despite her pioneering beginnings, leads a truly regular life, at
least when viewed externally. Ms. Brown, who turns thirty in
July 2008, is a postal worker in Bristol, England, who loves her
parents and shies away from public attention regarding her vit-
reous beginnings.

This, then, is a collective story, no matter how it turns out
individually: whether resulting in no live birth, one precious
singleton, or telltale multiples, whether necessitating repeated
attempts or science fiction–like variations on the basic procedure, these are the issues that we need negotiate even as we
profit by science.

When
Oligomenorrhea
Met Oligozoospermia

The website's wallpaper shows a shadowy baby blinking his shiny eyes once every second or so. Same sepia tone as my grandparents' wedding photo, sandwiched between diplomas in my home office. The fertility center's demo baby is too flat, with eyes glassier than a real child's. Same thing with my grandfather Max, who stares dead straight and unsmiling at one of those hulking 1930s camera lenses, despite the fact of his wedding day, his natty tuxedo and slick, precision-parted hair, his youth, and my unbelievably young grandmother, whose gauzy, tiered dress he'll presumably slip off later that day.

My grandmother, whose name was Mary but whom we all called Nanny, sits erect in a chair in front of Max, a gigantic floral arrangement suspended at knee level as a symbol of their cultivation, her fertility, a woman in bloom. She wears a flowing lace bonnet-cum-veil that someone—the photographer's assistant or perhaps a bridesmaid, my Aunt Pearl or Aunt Vivian—has swirled in a pool around her feet. Her mouth is clamped shut in an antismile as if Pearl, Vivian, or the photographer's assistant has warned her that only desperate women and greenhorns broadcast their marriage-day excitement.

The fertility baby's mouth is soft, and his fleshy lower lip gently glows, the indentation above his mouth a chiaroscurist's masterwork. An unseen light source illuminates his right ear, and my whispered wish for a child flies toward it. A block of text to the left welcomes me to the Reproductive Endocrinology Clinic. REC *offers all the advantages of a full-service, state-of-the-art reproductive center,* it promises, *while maintaining a warm and personable atmosphere.* I'm interested in knowing about the state of the art, but that baby is so distracting.

Some of the text bleeds over onto the baby and into his ear. The words *warm* and *helping* filter inside it like reassurances, a promise to this archetype that no matter how things turn out for him, no matter if the technology dooms him to ill health or unfit parents, the REC's intentions are beyond noble. They are munificent, civilized. They are humane.

The left ear lies in shadow, an elusive anatomical structure suggesting the abstract babies made tangible if only I click on the "Contact Us" prompt. Before committing myself, I look for signs that this is the sort of place with which Gary and I would want, or tolerate, intimate contact. I don't even mind so much the Wellesley, Massachusetts, location, approximately eight hundred impractical miles from my home in Chicago. I have friends who've traveled to New York to have squirts of their husband's blood shot into their own systems to try to overcome diagnosed allergies to spousal genetic material, and other friends who have trekked to orphanages in the shadow of Russian mountain ranges. So what's a few hundred miles for my own familiar child?

I examine Max and Nanny's picture for signs of the life they're to lead. They will have four children, my father the youngest, and all will be successful, by both immigrant and American standards. Obedient, handsome kids who master the piano, pose for family photos in coordinating sailors' outfits, and matriculate at good colleges. Max will die at eighty-one from a leukemia–skin cancer combination. Nanny will lead her life ashamed of her thickly accented English and lack of formal education. But she'll persevere, hosting brunches for her children and their grandchildren even as lung disease forces her to expectorate into plastic cottage cheese cartons scattered around tables in her condo.

The double-chinned baby's hair sticks up in feathery tufts. He has cowlicks, just like any old baby, convincing me that this process isn't about eugenics. It's about creating people who resemble their naturally conceived counterparts, down not only to the last hair but also to its complex follicular patterning. I wonder whether the REC baby will fare as well as my grandparents, all three of them plunked down in novel territory. Will he, like Nanny, feel shame in having come from a different place? His birth similar to the other guys in his kindergarten class, his conception something else altogether. Will vestiges of his earliest beginnings haunt him until his death, as they did her? Nanny's lung disease was a probable result of the typhus she suffered on the packed railcar that took her out of her village and into the subhuman conditions of the Minsk ghetto, where she stayed until her father, living with an uncle in Pittsburgh, earned enough money to send for his wife and children. Perhaps he'll end up, eighty years down the road, with an IVF-related cancer or a profound sense of alienation.

He's as cultivated as Nanny's bridal bouquet, further proof of the human quest to tame nature. Scientists have been successfully developing embryos in test tubes since the late 1970s. In the intervening years, a million more IVF children have quietly joined Louise Brown's ranks, substantiating the technology and proving themselves, like all beautiful babies, terrific marketing tools, just like the Goodyear tire–ensconced chubster, or the perfectly adorable preemie sleeping comfortably in an incubator brought to you by the Plastics Council.

That IVF baby's computerized blinking seems too aggressive, however, a look-at-me, want-me tactic when chubby thighs would suffice.

Baby blinks away while I read what the Reproductive Endocrinology Center has to offer.

What We Do. *Blink.* Our Pregnancy Rates. *Blink.* Insurance. *Blink.*

Come and meet one of our world class fertility expert for a free consultation.

There's a typo, *expert* without an *s*, one picayune omission but enough to confirm I'll have to seek my progeny elsewhere. When dealing with things microscopic—egg nuclei and isolated sperm—there can be no margin for error. Or maybe the REC does have only one expert, some one-scientist band with all the know-how. Not only does he harvest the eggs and evaluate cellular quality, he answers the phones, writes the brochures, and makes the baby blink. He's created this website as a flashy front to promote his rinky-dink operation as a professional, cutting-edge, high-tech facility with limitless capacity for helping the nonproofreading parent-hopeful reach her potential.

I've arrived at this particular website and somewhat agonizing juncture following two months of medical tests to explain health issues that I'd ignored until I decided I wanted to be pregnant. I saw my gynecologist, an elderly gentleman whose name I got from the receptionist at my office when I realized I had lived in Chicago for almost two years and hadn't had a checkup. He examined me and took my history.

I told Dr. Carter that in the past few years my periods had become irregular, bordering on nonexistent. I expressed my distress at having gained weight suddenly and without good explanation. In a matter of months I'd loaded ten pounds onto my smallish frame without so much as ingesting French-fried or frosted anything. In fact, I was training for a marathon, clocking sixty-plus miles a week and watching a nontraining husband carbo-load while I nibbled on sensible portions of lean proteins and leafy greens. Yet the weight crept up, morphing my previously toned upper arms and thighs and muscular belly into somebody else's, some potato-gorging couch dweller's physique.

And to make matters worse, my twenty-nine-year-old, and therefore completely mature, feet had grown. Like the bulk of my wardrobe, even my stretchiest, most worn-in shoes now felt tight. Dr. Carter took note of the bodily and podiatric expansion, the lack of periods, and my additional complaints of a rash-inducing intolerance to heat. He suggested I call his friend and colleague Dr. Peter Frankfurth, who specialized in reproductive endocrinology.

Unlike any other doctor I'd called for an appointment, Dr. Frankfurth had the receptionist transfer my call to his office.

"Hello, Elizabeth. This is Dr. Peter Frankfurth." He spoke slowly. "Dr. Carter told me you'd phone."

I had left Dr. Carter less than two hours ago, and Dr. Frankfurth had already heard from him? Had Dr. Carter called to marvel at my freakish symptoms and warn that he'd sent over a doozy? Was that even professional?

"Great man, very good doctor. So, could you be here tomorrow around two?"

Hanging up, I worried. Who but the very sickest of sick people got such full medical attention? I showed up the following afternoon, quietly said my name to the receptionist, and found my way over to a scratchy, tweedy sofa. The waiting area was paneled in imitation wood, the kind that is supposed to look real but if you keep looking at it shows the same exact wormhole constellations at even intervals; it should have belonged to a family doctor in Anchorage, circa 1950, and not to a late-twentieth-century endocrinologist. Nubby furniture and blobby oil paintings of fishing boats at sunset belonged to wellness-checking, strep-throat-swabbing general practitioners, the sort of doctors who looked after your whole person, from the top of your aching head to the bottoms of your athlete's feet.

Not that I'd ever been to any specialists—beyond pediatricians, gynecologists, and dentists, that is. I'd had an uneventful childhood medicine-wise, suffering only the occasional sprained wrist or ankle—standard gymnastics and kick-the-can injuries. But a doctor who investigated glands and hormones and lymph nodes required a space more august. It ought to have been whiter and less textured, a vague hint of bleach in the air, and lots of chrome light fixtures and surgical props for reflecting a patient's screaming-red shirt back at her.

Dusty magazines nestled in an oxidized brass basket-weave rack with loose, yellowed subscription cards and half-used legal pads. For several moments I seriously considered taking my business, whatever it proved to be, elsewhere, somewhere clearly sterile and that communicated that the principals understood that when dealing with particles and microns, only wipeable upholstery should be considered for the office furnishings. More to the point, when confronting a potentially serious health issue, this patient just plain doesn't want a too-comfy-looking specialist's office. It sends the scary message that Dr. Terminal is trying too hard to provide succor by way of easy chairs and nature paintings. He's reminding us of our human condition, that damned mortal coil, and that horrific maladies are just as much a part of the deal as fake wood paneling, magnificent sunsets, and magazines nobody wants to read. And those sun paintings! The four thick canvases with gonzo sunsets over bodies of water were credited to an artist named Manetta, who'd only half painted the sun, the horizon, the boats, concentrating the bulk of his effort, and tube upon tube of pigment, on making the reflections sing. The orange sun reflected as neon pink. A lone boat, standard-issue brown, was either halfway rotten or constructed by a boat builder with little regard for the importance of watertightness. The quadtych was a dirge reminding Dr. Frankfurth's patients that there is beauty beyond one's physical boundaries.

A man wearing Buddy Holly spectacles and a light blue exam coat with Peter Frankfurth M.D. embroidered in a looping script above a Northwestern University Medical Center badge opened a door into the waiting area and, confirming my name, asked me to please follow him. He walked slowly down the hall, his back to me the whole way, and I tried hard to slow my naturally quick pace lest I give him a flat tire. Once we reached the examination room, he asked me if I wouldn't mind terribly removing all my clothes, undergarments included, even though regular doctors let you keep your bra and socks on, and change into a gown with the opening in front. He seemed uncomfortable, like I was his very first patient, or like we were on a first date.

I'd barely finished tucking my gown beneath my legs on the paper-topped exam table when he knocked on the door and asked if I was ready. Then he put me through a series of unfamiliar tests. First he passed a magnifying glass slowly over my face, concentrating especially on the area surrounding my mouth. He pressed his own face so close to mine, I doubted whether he grasped the principle of magnification.

"Have you had a problem with hirsutism?" he asked, his breath warm on my cheek.

"As in excessive hair?" I asked, now certain the appointment would be even worse than I'd assumed.

"Yes. Any experience with excessive hair, you know, other than the soft, vellus hair normally present in females? Especially here?" He used his thumb to draw an invisible line across my jawbone. "Or here?" He backed away a couple of inches and massaged his own chin to indicate where my goatee might grow.

"No," I said. "I'm a little fuzzy, I guess. But so are most of the women in my family. It's pretty blonde. And I only ever notice it in direct sunlight. Like when I'm driving and happen to catch my reflection in my rolled-up window. What did you call that? Vellus?"

"Yes. Okay. Fine," Dr. Frankfurth said. "Please lie back." My gown crinkled as he spread it apart. "The following exam will feel a bit strange. It will be uncomfortable, to be certain, but it is central to my examination and, fortunately, quite brief. Or at least that's how it strikes me."

He stretched his hands out, fingers straight and rigid as an Olympic diver's, ta-dah! He vised first one and then the other of my nipples between his pointer fingers to see if he could manually extract liquid, "an indication of disorder in the non-lactating patient." He went to a sink in the corner of the room and squirted about six pumps of soap onto his hands, which I took as a sort of insult, turned on the water using a foot pedal, and began peppering me with questions.

"So, how would you describe your menstrual periods?" he asked.

I fixed my eyes on the stucco-looking ceiling panels, looking for familiar shapes among the meringuelike points. "I don't have them, really."

"No periods at all?" he followed up. "Or just irregular?"

"I have them occasionally, and even then I don't really bleed that much or for that long."

"Onset of menses?" he inquired.

"Thirteen," I said. I remember this because it was a couple of days after my bat mitzvah, a fact my mother trotted out as proof of God's existence.

"Fine. What about body odor?"

"Body odor? What do you mean?" I asked, finding a stucco terrier next to an old-fashioned stucco schoolhouse.

"Have you noticed any body odor?"

"On other people, yes. On myself, never. Although I use deodorant."

"What about coarse chest or facial hair? You said you were fuzzy. Does this term include any dark, wiry growth? Even one or two strands here or there?"

"No. Never," I said.

He weighed me, palpated my toe knuckles, and concluded that, if not for the growth of my feet, he'd assume I had a reproductive disorder. But the foot growth had him stumped. He drew several vials of blood and told me to make an appointment for the next week.

Midweek Dr. Frankfurth called me at work and asked if I could return later that day.

"So soon?" I asked, hoping he'd lost track of time. Daisy Johansen, the older lady who sat at the desk next to mine and who had complained during a staff retreat that "Beth broadcasts her personal business, her social plans, and her uninteresting opinions on the phone all day long while others in the office are trying to get work done," glanced up from the *Sun-Times* to glare at me.

"I'd like to chat about a possibility, and if you have the time now, I'd prefer not to wait. My last scheduled patient is at four. Could you be here this evening, say around five?"

I left work early, and for the first time, when I told my boss it was due to a medical emergency, I was telling the truth. Dr. Frankfurth was waiting in the reception area.

"Hello, Elizabeth," he said, handing me a dark gray three-ring binder with a square cartoon taped to its front. "I wanted to give you a chance to read through this while I finish up some paperwork. I'll see you in about ten minutes."

I sat down and remembered Dr. Frankfurth's stiff hands on my breasts. I couldn't shake the vision of him looking at my body, his greased-down wisps of hair striping his forehead like war paint.

I focused on the contents of the binder he'd handed me. Page after laminated page of cartoon doctor-patient interactions in examining rooms or sitting on either side of the doctor's peninsula of a partner's desk. In each, the doctor was either preparing to deliver, was delivering, or had just delivered bad news. The tiny, typed punchlines pointed to bright sides, the fact of both good and bad news, the importance that the patient pay immediately for services rendered.

Who would find this stuff funny? Maybe perfectly healthy people, people who didn't have Sasquatch feet all of a sudden, that's who. Or maybe this was just the thing to tickle fatally ill believers in a smashing afterlife. *Did you see this one?* a hospice care inmate asks over the hiss of his ventilator. *The doctor wants this pale, sore-covered fellow to make sure and pay his bill on his way out. That's rich.*

Dr. Frankfurth said my name and then cleared his throat. Clutching the binder, I followed him down the wood-paneled hallway, into his office, and onto a guest chair exactly like those I'd seen in the comics.

"Well, I've discussed your case with a few colleagues, and we all think this might be a hypothalamic tumor. No other diagnosis explains your array of symptoms. You see, in simple cases of hormone imbalance, we do expect to see some of your issues, the weight gain and lack of menstruation in particular. But its sudden onset and the fact you lack other telltale symptoms—no hirsutism, and as far as I'm concerned, you're really not clinically overweight, only heavier than you'd like to see yourself—point to something else. What really troubles me in particular is the foot growth. It can be a real tip-off. So yes, I'm comfortable saying this is most likely a hypothalamic tumor."

I knew the hypothalamus was located at the base of the brain, and I definitely knew the relationship between tumors and cancer. I was stunned. Done for at age twenty-nine, despite my healthy habits and my familial longevity, my great-grandmother Bubbe, who lived to be one hundred and something, and my grandparents who, if not for sun-worshipping, smoking, exposure to environmental toxins in their youth, and a diet rich in chopped liver, could have lived even longer than that. I was a runner, a non–meat eater, a lard-avoiding subscriber to *Vegetarian Times*. I didn't smoke, hardly ever drank, and then only red wine and beer, arguably healthful beverages.

"Let me continue," Dr. Frankfurth said. "These sorts of tumors are generally operable and responsive to radiation or chemotherapy or some combination thereof. The treatment will depend on the aggressiveness of the tumor and whether it's a glioma or another type of cancer, if cancer at all, of course."

"So it's not necessarily cancer?" I asked, not yet crying but not exactly not crying, either.

"Maybe, maybe not. But if it is, special radiation treatments can be focused on some tumors and can be as effective as surgery, with less risk to surrounding tissue. Brain swelling caused by a tumor may need to be treated with steroids. We'll also probably need to correct what I presume to be hormone imbalances through hormone replacement or suppression. Of course we still have to substantiate the diagnosis with some high-resonance imaging."

Dr. Frankfurth wrote out a requisition for an MRI place a couple of floors down in the same office building. He described a couple of top-notch neurosurgical practices, one in Detroit, the other in Palo Alto, in case radiation didn't succeed or was deemed the incorrect protocol. Then he handed me some literature, a paper booklet called "Hypothalamic Glioma." It had a line drawing of a white woman and a black man hugging on its cover.

When he saw I had finished reading, a determination made from the lowered brochure and the shaking hand slapped over my gaping mouth, Dr. Frankfurth reminded me that we still needed to wait for the blood-test results to return three days hence. He cautioned me, however, that his conferences with colleagues pointed strongly to a tumor that caused me to produce an excess of male hormones—some combination of testosterone and androgens. The pressure of the tumor on my hypothalamus, he deduced, was what had caused the foot growth.

As I drove home, I decided not to phone Gary. In the first place, I didn't want him to worry needlessly. I was having an MRI the next day, and couldn't I hold out until confirmation? Second, and more to the point, I didn't want to use my cell phone. Maybe *it* had caused the tumor, its cellular waves beaming into my brain and monkeying with its cellular structure. A Motorolymphoma taking up residence in the base of my head, proof that, as Nanny liked to remind me, the technology my generation took for granted would one day kill us. She invoked my brother's friend, a woman in her early twenties who'd been forced at gunpoint to withdraw money at an ATM and then taken to an alley and shot execution style. I could hear Nanny making clear the similarity between my situation and this girl's, a fatal wound to the head delivered not with a gun but with a cellular phone, the sound of gunshot replaced with the ringing sound of Beethoven's Fifth.

Unable to ignore technology completely, I went online upon returning home, a trek that involved alternating fits of crying and singing along with a lite-FM station, a reminder of the good old days and proof that no matter how big the tumor, it hadn't yet affected the portion of my brain storing the Journey lyrics.

I Googled some of my newly acquired lingo. *Glioma* yielded numerous sites. The first, gliomas.com, told me there is *new hope for patients with brain tumors.* Wasn't *hope* a term defying qualification? *New hope,* two little words, and I realized that my diagnosis had placed me in the stream of an ongoing, terrible situation—like category-five rapids. But at least I'd entered them at a time when improvements had been made to the leaky lifeboats and patched helmets.

Gliomas.com let me know that *malignant brain tumors (gliomas) are rarely cured by surgery and/or radiotherapy alone.*

Chemotherapy, as generally available, has been of limited value. As generally available? I smelled a pitch coming on. I kept reading, situated smack dab as I was in the middle of the target audience.

> Dr. Isaac Djerassi has perfected a form of intensive chemotherapy which is proving to be the most effective treatment for brain gliomas. Among 200 patients with brain glioma, treated by his method, 70% have shown substantial reduction or disappearance of their tumors, with marked improvement of their symptoms and prolonged survival. Eighteen of 57 (31%) patients with advanced and terminal Grade III or near Grade III Glioblastoma were alive at 10 to 28 years with a median of over 10 years . . . Higher success rates are expected in recently diagnosed and previously untreated patients in good general condition.

I examined the stats and felt not relieved but sick, in the way *sick* had previously meant, like my stomach had taken over my heart and both were making themselves felt at the back of my throat.

> The existence of this site is not an attempt to practice medicine.
> Use of the site does not establish a doctor-patient relationship.
> Consult a qualified health care provider for medical advice . . .
> We reserve the right to change its disclaimer and all other terms and policies, so users should review these periodically.

Hey, hospice care patient. You hear that? Please make certain to review the disclaimer, terms, and policies on your way out.

Other glioma sites had hyperlinks to support groups and chat rooms where patients shared their experiences, mostly not good, and family members memorialized their beloved, dearly departed ones, consistently so not good.

The next day I went for my MRI. With my head tightly Velcroed still within the imaging machine, a vanilla-colored ellipse with a sliding pallet upon which I was to lie perfectly motionless, I asked the technician if she saw anything scary.

"I can't tell you that, even if I did see something," she said, making clear she wasn't in the mood for chitchat.

I parsed her comment for hints. I decided the word *even* meant she didn't see anything. Or maybe she just sucked at her job, and a good MRI technician would see lots of disturbing stuff: tumors, fissures in my cranium, perhaps a shriveled lobe or two. When she had finished, she told me I could leave without stopping at the front desk. They'd send the results directly to my physician.

After what felt like forever—you'd think I'd have a new hyperawareness of time as a too-fleeting luxury—but was really only three days, Dr. Frankfurth called.

"I received the imaging and the results of your complete blood workup. I am ever so happy to report, young lady, that I have good news. While you do have a condition, it is somewhat common and definitely manageable. It's something called Polycystic Ovarian Syndrome or PCOD, for Polycystic Ovarian Disorder, and it's something your regular obstetrician can help you manage. The only thing I can't figure out is the foot growth. But I suppose with your excessive running, it isn't impossible that there's been some swelling, flattening, and possibly some bone shifting."

Dr. Frankfurth had referred to my problem alternately as a syndrome and a disorder, so I'm not sure which it was, or if it mattered, although *disorder* sounded less serious, something slightly off, like a bumped checkerboard.

"There may be anywhere between six and ten million

women in the U.S. with PCOD," Dr. Frankfurth had told me by way of comfort. "I know that's hardly a dead-on statistic, but the trouble with this condition is its resemblance to other things."

"Like brain tumors?" I asked.

"In your case, yes. But many women just chalk up their hardly desirous symptoms to excessively active sebaceous glands, a sedentary lifestyle, or a sweet tooth. Most women we see with PCOD have acne across their jaw lines, more facial hair than would be typical for females, and fairly significant weight problems. Still others, such as you, have a pinch of this symptom, a trace of that. Hence the difficulty of absolute diagnosis. However, in your case, I stand behind my findings. Your menstrual history and blood results—and let's not forget your weight gain, and the fact that it most definitely is not a hypothalamic tumor—make it fairly certain." Dr. Frankfurth suggested I follow up with Dr. Carter and get his recommendations for conception, if that was something I was still interested in.

Dr. Carter confirmed that between 3 and 5 percent of all women have PCOD and that for many of them getting pregnant is tricky since ovulation occurs irregularly if at all. He explained that an overabundance of the male hormone androgen causes the hairiness, but since I wasn't noticeably hairy (making me not hairy, right?), my androgen level was probably not especially elevated. He recommended I make an appointment for a pelvic ultrasound to check for follicular clusters in each ovary and that since I worked in the same building as one of the area's largest fertility clinics, the Human Reproduction Institute (HRI), the very place whose name on the elevator directory caused me to envision daily a vast, pulsing orgy, I should be seen there.

Gary and I decided to go to this next appointment together.

He waited in the reception area while I underwent a pelvic ultrasound. Test completed and pants pulled back up, I met Gary in reception, where we sat and listened to the receptionist on the phone. She spoke in a regular, nonquiet voice of a third party whom she alternately referred to as "that bitch" and "that whore." Finally a woman appeared from behind a swinging door into another part of the office and asked us to follow her. "You'll be seeing Dr. Lomas," she said. "You're lucky. He's excellent."

Dr. Lomas was seated behind his desk, his window treatments drawn all the way to the ceiling, letting in the sunlight and a spectacular view straight down Michigan Avenue. I looked at the buildings and the bridge, the buses, cars, cabs, and sidewalks teeming with people and their normally functioning reproductive systems. Dr. Lomas flipped through papers, took a couple of notes on a small pad next to the stack. He hadn't looked up since we'd entered.

"Well," he said, smoothing the papers and focusing on Gary. "Your wife has polycystic ovaries. Has this condition been explained to you?"

"To me?" Gary asked.

"PCO, or polycystic ovaries, mean there are many cysts, or follicles, in each ovary. So many follicles in your ovaries," Dr. Lomas continued, shifting his attention to me, "that there is very little chance you'll ever produce enough hormone in any particular month to spur a follicle to maturation sufficient for ovulation to occur. My strong recommendation is to start you on clomiphene citrate, Clomid as it is commonly known, to help your ovaries develop more dominant eggs. What happens is, the Clomid tricks your system into thinking it's not making enough estrogen, causing your hypothalamus to release gonadotropin-releasing hormone, or GnRH, which stimulates the release of follicle-stimulating hormone, FSH, into your bloodstream. In turn, the FSH stimulates the ovary into estrogen production, causing follicular growth. Eighty percent of women taking clomiphene citrate end up ovulating. I'll have you keep detailed records of your sexual activity so that we may ascertain whether you are having ample intercourse for a pregnancy to result. Also, since your blood test showed high levels of luteinizing hormone, also known as LH, in ratio to follicle-stimulating hormone, which I've already told you is referred to as FSH, I'm recommending that before we begin Clomid, we normalize your system by putting you on a birth control pill for a couple of months. We'll take you off, wait a couple more months, and then we'll be set to try the Clomid."

I'd never felt more impatient. I was anxious for pregnancy and not so thrilled by how long it might take. Doing the math, I realized that I wouldn't even start fertility medication for four months. Even if I got pregnant within days of starting the Clomid, it'd be over a year before I'd lay eyes on my baby.

Unenthusiastically, I filled the prescriptions, swallowed a birth control pill daily for two months, then went off the pill for two months and began taking one Clomid a day. Clomid! At long last! I finally felt reproductive, like I was doing the things people do when they need that little nudge in the fertility department.

After wavering between a simple diary and an actual chart to note Gary's and my sexual activity and deciding Dr. Lomas seemed more like a chart guy, I grabbed a ruler and a pencil and began laying out my graph. I found myself blinking, rubbing my eyes. The lines on the paper flickered. Standing up and looking around the kitchen, I realized my vision was blurry. I called HRI and told the receptionist I was a patient of Dr. Lomas's and that I thought I was having a bad reaction to the Clomid.

"Hold on," the receptionist said. I held for upward of five minutes before hanging up. I called again and once again explained to the receptionist who I was and what was going on and that I was worried. "Hold on," she said again, and again I held. Just as I was about to hang up, somebody answered and told me she was Dr. Lomas's nurse.

"My name is Elizabeth Kohl Feinerman, and I'm worried about how the Clomid is making me feel," I told her.

"What's your chart number?" she asked.

"I don't know. But I'm a patient of Dr. Lomas's and I started my Clomid, and all of a sudden my vision is completely blurred. Is this normal?"

"I really need your chart number," she said. "Then I'll be able to answer your questions."

I hadn't memorized my chart number, and my vision was so bad that the thought of looking through the HRI folder made me queasy. "I don't have it, and I'm not able to see clearly so even if I could find it, I don't think I could read it."

"What I can tell you—but I must warn that without know-ing your medical information or the underlying cause of your infertility and am only offering general information—is that in some instances blurring of the vision can occur. It's because your body has been tricked into thinking it doesn't have enough estrogen, so you experience menopausal symptoms: nausea, hot flashes, headaches, and blurred vision among them. Oh. I just found your chart. Just a minute."

I heard paper noises.

"Why would Dr. Lomas have put you on Clomid?" she asked.

"I don't know. To help my ovaries?"

"Your ovaries have way too many follicles in them. I think Clomid is dangerous for you. You could hyperstimulate and end up hospitalized, minus one ovary that got so heavy with follicles that it twisted on its fallopian tube stem and became damaged beyond repair. I am not authorized to override Dr. Lo-mas's orders, but let me talk to him about you. In the meantime keep taking the Clomid until you hear back from us."

I stopped taking the Clomid. When Dr. Lomas's nurse called back the next day with information, I told her that's okay, I had decided not to treat my infertility at their center, thanks anyway. "Good luck," she said as if she really meant it. "And don't you dare let any other doctors put you on Clomid. It could ruin any chance you have of ever giving birth."

Dr. Bhavana Paswan's waiting room featured still-life watercolors signed by the artist, Bhavana Paswan. At last, I thought, a creative and artistic doctor, somebody who'll consider me an individual and not some chart number. Or perhaps she keeps track of her patients using another, more inventive sorting technique. Like parking structures that assign a local sports team or architectural highlight to each floor to help people remember where they parked, perhaps Dr. Paswan would examine my multifollicular ovaries and categorize me as "Seurat."

"Look, Gary," I said, pointing to a painting of a squash on a yellow dish, "this is by Dr. Paswan."

"Oh," he said, sitting down and grabbing a copy of *Mother Jones.*

The receptionist inquired whether we'd like anything to drink. Filtered water or herbal tea, perhaps?

"I'd love some coffee," Gary said. The receptionist wagged her finger.

"No coffee. Dr. Paswan believes the chemicals in coffee cause cancer. And no caffeine either. It kills sperm."

"Nothing. Thank you," Gary said.

We waited for a bit; then a short, colorfully dressed woman holding hands with a woman I actually knew emerged through that door that all doctors apparently have separating the waiting area from the exam rooms and offices. The woman I knew was crying, and Dr. Paswan was squeezing her hand. "Be patient," Dr. Paswan said. She had a thick accent. "It's too soon."

The woman I knew looked up at me, smiled a little as if she recognized me, too, then left.

"Well, you must be Elizabeth and Gary," Dr. Paswan said,

extending her hand. "I am Dr. Paswan and this is my pleasure and privilege. Please come with me. I'd like to have a talk and see what I can do for you."

I was psyched. Dr. Paswan was warm and sweet, and I felt good about my chances with her. She'd know better than to prescribe the wrong drugs, and she'd be sensitive to my need, my intense desire not to wait for months even to begin trying. She looked like a mom, so she'd get the whole instinct thing. And the truth was, at this point, my maternal instinct was surging and poised to do battle with any obstacles that got in its way.

"Elizabeth and Gary, I read the information you had sent over. I thank you for doing so. The first thing I want to say is that I believe you have been misdiagnosed, my dear."

"What?" I said.

Gary pulled my sleeve a little, and I leaned in. "I don't understand her," he whispered. Gary has trouble understanding accented English. He was in England once and struggled to get around, due to the language barrier.

"And Elizabeth, when we spoke on the phone, I could hear in your voice instantly that you are what they call a type A personality. In my experience, women with this personality characteristic can have tremendous problems with their fertility if they don't do anything to stem it. What I strongly suspect, my dear, is that your body is in a state of hysterical infertility, and that once we can get you to relax and detox, things will function normally and beautifully. Your constant stress level wrecks hormonal balance. We'll fix that. Gary?"

I tapped Gary with my shoe, so he'd know she was talking to him.

"What type of undergarments do you wear?"

"Pardon me?" he asked.

"Do you wear cotton underpants, my dear?"

"He wears boxer shorts," I answered. "Gary has a little trouble understanding your accent, I think."

"Is this true?" Dr. Paswan asked Gary.

"Yes. Boxers. I always wore them, and our doctor at HRI said they're good since they keep everything cool."

"Bullshit!" Paswan said hostilely. "That is typical Western-style BS. One of my interests is the relationship between the environment, including the fabrics we wear, the sheets we sleep on, and the couches we occupy, and the anatomy. What you must remember is that while it is simple to have stylish clothes and fashionable waterproof sofas, what does that matter when your wrinkle-free, stain-resistant fashions cause disease in the body? Did you know that the chemicals in your clothing can and do cause your body to shut down? Maybe not all at once. But a few thousand sperm here and a few thousand sperm there, and pretty soon, as Illinois's own Senator Dirksen once said, we're talking about real sperm damage."

We left Dr. Paswan's with a copy of her paper, "Environmental Chemicals and the Body," thereafter referred to by Gary as "PCBs in Your Pants." There were also a few printouts suggesting "The Optimal Diet for Reproductive and Nonreproductive Health" and highlighted points from A *Chakra and Kundalini Workbook: Psycho-Spiritual Techniques for Health, Rejuvenation and Reproduction.*

I had been told that, besides caffeine, I was not to ingest saccharine, white flour, cornstarch, white potatoes, or carbonated anything. Dr. Paswan suggested that we not only cease using our microwave but get rid of it altogether. "It constantly leaks harmful rays, even when off. The plastics they use not only leach their own deadly chemicals into the air, but they act like a slow-release sponge for the microwaves. Nasty, terrible things. They should be outlawed."

I was cautioned to stop running and take up swimming, with instructions to try to conjure, while submerged, my earliest beginnings in the watery peace of my mother's womb. "Get the head right, and the uterus will follow," Dr. Paswan explained. "Identify with the baby you seek, and a cellular shift will occur, yielding a more hospitable environment for pregnancy."

It was suggested that once Gary changed his underwear to those made from 100 percent organic cotton, "roomy enough not to stifle his organic function, but not so loose that they didn't gently cradle the testes," Dr. Paswan wouldn't need to see him again. As for me, I was to begin these pragmatic changes and check in twice weekly for chats and so that she could check my epidermis—particularly along my jawline and upper arms, where I tended toward ruddiness—for change. Once she sensed sufficient evolution, she'd perform an ultrasound to ensure that my ovaries reflected my new and improved personality. Oh, and by the way, she didn't perform the IVF herself, only the ultrasounds and blood tests and, most important, the psychological and spiritual adjustments. For the IVF, she contracted with another doctor to whom she said she'd introduce us when she determined we were ready.

A couple of weeks later, while in the health club locker room following a very chilly, crowded, and unwomblike swim, I overheard two women talking.

"Oh my God!" one of them squealed. "You're pregnant. Please tell me you're pregnant. I'll feel so bad if I said that and you're not."

"Four months," the apparently pregnant one replied.

"You look great. I mean for someone who is pregnant. I'm so happy for you guys."

"Me too. It was such a to-do. We tried for a couple of years, which is no fun after about the first month, having to have all this sex you're not into and month after month of having nothing happen, even though I am totally regular and was pregnant twice before, you know before I was married. So anyway, we went to this doctor a few people I knew raved about, and they were right, he's great. First of all, not that it matters, but he's kind of hot. Sexy in an unobvious way, you know? He's one of those guys whose niceness makes them good-looking, but not so obviously hot that I felt uncomfortable or my husband would even think of it. Just the perfect amount for a doctor. And Mark really likes him, too, which is a minor miracle."

"I didn't realize you were having problems. Why didn't you say anything?"

"Believe me, it's not the kind of thing you want to talk about. And even though Dr. Hamlin, that doctor—you may have actually seen him working out here, he's always running on the treadmill—anyway, even though I thought it'd probably work since just about everybody who goes to him ends up with a baby, of their own I mean, I just didn't want to jinx it. You know? And me, too, in about five months."

"I'm thrilled for you guys," the other woman said, turning on the blow dryer. "And you look really beautiful!" she yelled over the hum. "Your boobs are so huge. I hope when I get pregnant I'll look like that!"

The first thing Dr. Hamlin's clinic, Great Lakes Fertility, required was that we attend an introductory seminar. The moderator, an infertility-treatment psychologist named Cara Alberts, kicked off her talk with some hard facts. I scanned the room, checking out the audience, as Cara began.

"Good evening. Before you and your partner begin your treatment, you should know that in vitro fertilization is emotionally and psychologically stressful. The treatment program is very time-consuming and disruptive to people's lives. But you should also know that infertility is a part of the human condition and that you're not alone. In fact, it affects anywhere between ten and fifteen percent of any population. And luckily we live in a time where, difficult as it can be, treatment does exist."

Eight other couples plus two unaccompanied women—one

who looked forty or so, the other wearing a Blackhawks jersey and a ponytail jacked on the side of her head—watched as Cara Alberts flicked on a slide projector and pivoted to face a portable movie screen beside the podium.

"Hormone injections," she said. She slapped the projected word with the back of her open hand. "Numerous appointments to monitor progress. Egg retrieval and embryo transfer procedures." She advanced the slides, and we saw an illumined calculation.

Injections + Appointments + Egg Retrieval + Embryo Transfer = RESOURCES (energy × time × emotions)

"That's the most depressing story problem I've ever seen," I whispered to Gary. An East Indian couple two rows up turned around and the wife shushed me. Her husband shushed her and mouthed *sorry* to me. *It's all right,* I mouthed back. Gary shushed me.

"Is there a problem up there?" Cara Alberts stood in front of the screen, the word *Egg* writ in black light on her forehead. "Well then. I'm distributing an IVF preparation checklist. I'd like you and your partner to go through it, initial each item so that I'll know you've read and understand it, and hand it back to me on your way out this evening. I notice a couple of you don't have partners. We'll become quite familiar in the coming days and weeks. Please indicate at the top of your sheets, ladies, that you're alone."

She navigated the aisles, passing papers down each occupied row.

"One thing I forgot to mention," she said. She stood next to us, extending a handout toward Gary. "There is no guarantee of having an IVF cycle end in a pregnancy. On the average, only one in five completed IVF cycles will result in a baby."

"Great," Gary said, reaching toward the paper. "Thanks."

Cara Alberts handed him our checklist and walked up the rest of the steps and toward the auditorium door. She moved her suit jacket sleeve away from her wristwatch and, still looking at the watch, asked, "Are there any questions?"

At this point I had loads of questions. Still putting aside whether or not people should tamper with nature to this extent, I wondered whether kids who result not from ordinary sex (dimmed lights, R&B, orgasm) but from extraordinary feats of science (hysterosonogram, microdose Lupron, intracytoplasmic sperm injection) are completely normal. Are science-babies exactly like the traditional kind? Are they physical duplicates down to the last cell, atom, particle? If you gathered up the strands from a first haircut and arranged them under an electron microscope, could you detect a difference? The molecular sequence on the science-baby's hair too perfect, like an artist's rendering of hair in nature? What about health risks? Life expectancies? Hobbies? Interests?

Imaging

A twenty-four-mile stretch of beautified Illinois interstate separates the Fullerton on-ramp from the Highland Park exit-ramp. A Budweiser billboard digitally alternates between the time (5:51 a.m.) and the temperature (14 degrees Fahrenheit), reminding me I'd rather be in Cancún, drinking *cerveza* in a cabana overlooking an abandoned stretch of *playa*. Instead I'm on the Kennedy Expressway. The concrete-stalked street-lights—lined up on either side of the northbound lanes, their arched and funnel-tipped ends dangling opaque bulbs like an ovulation on steroids—switch abruptly off. The sun has risen, rendering this Chicago Public Works machinery sud-denly obsolete.

A nurse instructed me not to eat this morning, so of course I can think of nothing but food: bacon momentarily, then puffy spinach-filled omelets, and finally light brown air-pocked pan-cakes. Buttermilk blackberry. Chocolate chip short stacks. Buck-wheat half-dollars. Oh, the sounds of them, the variations!

Saturdays growing up, my mom made enough to feed not only the three kids she had but also the two miscarried others she quietly thanked God for displacing to make room for Danny, David, and me.

Mom would beat the batter in an aluminum bowl, her whisk whirling like a bionic appendage. She mixed rhythmically, each pass an audible scraping, the wiry cone cutting through the bubbling butter-yellow cream. After ladling one preparatory circle into the hot pan, she'd pronounce, "The first one is for practice," and inspect the edges for traces of smoke. "It's the same thing with kids," she'd say, forcing a spatula under the blackening tissue-thin sides of the virgin cake and flipping it into the garbage. "You make all your mistakes on the first and hope the rest turn out just right." David and I would scan our older brother Danny, searching for marks. We decided he was the only one our mom ever spanked with the back of a hairbrush because he was her starter kid.

I wonder, what if one kid is all there ever is? A lone lab rat forced to bear the brunt of his folks' novice parenting, one basket towering with all the genetic eggs? I also wonder what my mother would have done if she were Chinese, and, in accordance with China's family planning and population control policy, permitted only a child or two, depending on whether she lived in an urban or rural setting. Which would her freshly built French Provincial in a semirustic suburb classify as, and what would she have done with all the extra bedrooms, all that closet space? Certainly, in the shoes of a woman with restricted liberties, she'd find incomprehensible this uniquely American, baby-boomer construct of starters—starter house, starter job, starter marriage, starter child upon which to perfect one's parenting techniques.

Perhaps my mother would have joined all those Chinese women who aborted female fetuses, not wanting to waste their limited number of children on anything but the culturally favored boy. The whispered advice she routinely gave me,

"Whatever you do, have a daughter," a cruel wish for both mother and child when that baby could be killed or abandoned at birth, starved to death, sold, or left in a field to die, when that mother could be punished for her apparent inability to bear sons.

A 1998 article in London's *Daily Telegraph* about forced abortion and sterilization in the Huaiji region of China, an impoverished area 140 miles from Hong Kong, described a culture where boys are vastly preferred and technology is more commonly enlisted to prevent unwanted children (namely girls and disabled babies) than to help create them. Government officials acquire expensive ultrasound equipment to enforce family planning policies, driving the machines around to outlying villages, where local doctors force women of childbearing age to undergo tests. When a pregnancy is detected, the doctors perform an abortion on the spot, the ultrasound machine pushed aside to make room for an abortive saline injection. Even "heavily pregnant" women—up to eight and a half months—are forced to void babies in this way.

In Beijing, according to the People's Republic's 2001 census, the birth ratio of males to females has increased dramatically, a direct result of the use of ultrasound for gender selection. In 2000 over 116 male births were recorded for every 100 females, compared to a natural ratio of 106 males per 100 females, resulting in an estimated 70 million more males than females in China. And the U.S.-based Population and Development Review confirms widespread Chinese abuse of sonogram technology for sex selection. As female babies are born in lower numbers, there are reports of little girls being kidnapped or taken from one village to serve or marry in others, although female infanticide, the historical, low-tech method for sex selection, has become less common.

The perceived abuse of sonogram technology for abortive procedures is the reason, some experts say, that more funds have not gone toward easing the staggering rates of women dying in childbirth in developing countries. According to Nicholas Kristof, who wrote of maternal mortality in a 2006 *New York Times* op-ed, African women have a one-in-twenty chance of dying in pregnancy. Kristof writes that "in much of the world, the most dangerous thing a woman can do is to become pregnant." The problem is that, without the availability of emergency obstetric services, even small complications can prove fatal. The United Nations Population Fund, which addresses maternal mortality, no longer receives any U.S. funds since the Bush administration believes the agency supports abortions to control population in China.

In October 2005 the *Chicago Tribune* reported that relatives of pregnant Chinese peasants were being imprisoned to enforce the one-child rule. According to the article, family planning offices jail the families of peasants who go underground to duck unwanted medical procedures. A seventy-five-year-old man said he'd been detained for a month—a governmental tactic to pressure his pregnant daughter-in-law to emerge from hiding and have an abortion. Chen Guangcheng, a prominent activist in a town sixty miles northeast of Nigou, described the ongoing, aggressive campaign against the mostly peasant citizenry, despite a 2002 law barring officials from violating citizens' rights. Chen reported that in one rural county alone seven thousand people were sterilized between March and July 2005.

The *Daily Telegraph*'s online version, *Electronic Telegraph*, ran a story about a doctor, Gao Xiao Duan, who spent fourteen years as head of a "planned birth" office, a center established in Fujian province to enforce the one-child policy. She described how she escaped China with profound remorse for the harm she had done to women and their aborted children and a sense that there'd be international interest in this story. To that end, she'd smuggled out a videotape documenting the policy and its implementation.

Gao testified before Congress, and explained on *Nightline*, that women (even those nine months pregnant) involuntarily underwent abortion; others were forcibly sterilized; and those who flouted the one-child norm could and would have their houses burned down. She also described how detailed records of the marital, reproductive, and birth control history of every woman in town, down to the dates of her menstrual cycle, are itemized on a computer in a government office.

She related a terrible story about a nine-months-pregnant woman who was led out of an interview room and into an adjoining abortion room after her papers were examined and it came to light that she had unlawfully requested that "no birth certificate" be issued for her baby. Gao, and presumably the expectant mother, watched as the baby was taken from the woman's body. (It is unclear how this was accomplished.) As Gao describes it, "In the operating room, I saw how the aborted child's lips were sucking, how its limbs were stretching. A doctor injected poison into its skull, and the child died and was thrown in the trash can."

I can't imagine the horror of delivering a fully formed baby, not only to witness its murder at the hands of those who'd just delivered it, but to learn its features while watching it die. The bureaucratic and meticulous record-keeping about biological processes is something to which I can, however, relate: those detailed, pixilated charts, the decimal-pointed numbers inside brick-shaped boxes, all my ebbs and flows neatly organized into columns, tidy as a mathematical equation. And that deadpan question asked over and over, "First date of your last period?" and my unwavering, embarrassed, and increasingly exasperated response, "I don't get my period," noted somehow (a picture of a maxipad inside a circle with a hash mark drawn through it?) on a chart that grows thicker by the day. I wonder why they ask that same question each time, particularly in light of that hulking mass of paperwork they haul around, the one that ostensibly contains the nitty-gritty of my increasingly complicated medical history.

Do these nurses and lab technicians think I am holding out on them? That if they ask often enough, I will break down and admit that I *did* have my period, that it had started on the fifth of the month, a week ago last Thursday, in the middle of the afternoon while riding in an elevator? That I had experienced two days of heavy flow followed by a gradual tapering off for a total of six and a half days of menstruation? That I had employed nine tampons, six winged pads, ten tablets of Midol, three Hershey's kisses with almonds and seven without?

Like many patients before me, I worry what other information that chart might contain. In addition to all the medical data, vital statistics, and test results, are there subjective observations on the part of the doctors and nurses? *Mrs. Feinerman seems especially moody today. Mrs. Feinerman often wears frayed jeans and unfashionable sweater vests. Mrs. Feinerman certainly could use the name of my hair stylist/colorist.* Does the hard data they continue to compile point to some other conditions? Something medical and devastating but beyond the realm of their specialties and interests and therefore somebody else's fish to fry?

And what will be the ultimate fate of all of these written records? What if I run for political office and they are used against me somehow; could my heavy reliance on a plum insurance policy be considered proof that I don't truly believe in the universal health care plan upon which I'd built my platform? What if I become a famous actress and somebody sells them to Us *Weekly*, my fluctuating weight or atypical physique prompting an article on my real-life woes? Or what if I end up joining a nature commune, the Rainbow Family of Living Light or whatever it's called, and somebody figures out that my children, streamers in their long, unbrushed hair, dirt in their shoeless toes, aren't the same as all the other grimy kids? That they've been engineered, are the product of corrupt Western medical and consumer culture, their om-chanting mother just another mindless consumer of whatever new and shiny technology is dangled before her, Sister Sunshine nothing but a naïve and ignorant medication whore?

In 2002 *The New York Times* ran a story about fertility clinic ads for sex selection in newspapers catering to Indian expatriates in the United States and Canada. Indian feminists in the United States criticized the ads, laying out the skewed sex ratios in South and East Asia—experts estimate as many as 100 million "missing girls"—resulting from female infanticide, neglect of girl babies, and prenatal diagnosis leading to sex-selective abortion. The article reported that these ads would be illegal in India and that one of the publications dropped them as a result of the controversy.

The *New York Times* Sunday Styles section has run an ad for the Genetics & IVF Institute (GIVF), a Virginia-based fertility clinic with auxiliary locations in California, Minnesota, Texas, and China. The headline asks, "Do You Want to Choose the Gender of Your Next Baby?" The text answers that if so, you'd join "prospective parents from all over the world" who come to GIVF for an "exclusive scientifically-based sperm sorting gender selection procedure."

The preconception gender-selection procedure, known as MicroSort, is described as a means for selecting a boy or a girl for one of two purposes: either for the "prevention of genetic diseases" (by not choosing the sex affected by an X- or Y-linked condition) or for "family balancing" (selecting for a boy in a family that already has girls, or vice versa). "Family balancing," a term coined and popularized by GIVF's founder, Dr. Joseph Schulman, has been used since the early 1990s as justification for preconception gender selection.

Flow cytometric separated human sperm cells, or Micro-Sort, is a trademarked medical procedure, and the fact that

GIVF advertises it in *The New York Times*—as opposed to reaching potential consumers exclusively through targeted or discreet channels, online, or through medical networks—represents a striking and somewhat troubling relationship between a taboo social topic, medicine, and capitalism. Some bioethicists worry about creating consumer demand for still largely untested procedures. Others criticize MicroSort as a form of eugenics.

GIVF, sensitive to these charges, addressed the gender-discrimination issue on its website. The language used invokes American patriotism and traditional feminism, the phrases reverberating with echoes of the Constitution and the pro-choice movement.

> Fundamental principles of liberty affirm that couples should be free to choose their own reproductive options. The preferential conception of a daughter in couples at risk for transmitting an X-linked disease provides the couple a higher likelihood of an unaffected child. Furthermore, several surveys have indicated that a majority of couples approve in principle of preconception gender selection for purposes of family balancing (Rosenzweig and Adelman, 1976 and Markle and Nam, 1982). Our experience with couples who actually inquired about gender selection indicates that 53.6% of such inquirers desired female offspring. This slight preference for girls is consistent with other reports by Batzofin (1987) for American couples and Liu and Rose (1995) in Great Britain. The majority of couples (90.5%) in our study were seeking gender preselection for family balancing purposes, were in their mid 30's, had 2–3 children of the same sex, and desired only one more child.

The technology behind MicroSort was developed in the late 1980s by a government scientist at the U.S. Department of Agriculture for use in livestock reproduction. A couple of years later the USDA granted Dr. Schulman an exclusive U.S. license to apply the method to humans. The first MicroSort baby was born in 1995, and MicroSort now has established relationships with dozens of "physician collaborators" in the United States and "international collaborators" in seven other countries.

In 2001 the ASRM approved sperm sorting for "family balancing" after its ethics committee considered a range of potential social and ethical objections to it. The ASRM remains officially opposed to using preimplantation genetic diagnosis (PGD) for "family balancing," though in September 2001 its ethics committee chair, John Robertson, expressed in a letter a personal opinion at odds with the organization's opposition to PGD for sex selection.

In a *New York Times* article covering the chair's opinion, a fertility doctor wondered what would be the next step. Would learning more about genetics lead people to reject children who lack certain characteristics, like a particular IQ or hair or eye color? Feminists and other advocates for responsible uses of human genetic technologies also rallied against the apparent reversal, concerned that it was little more than consumer eugenics, in which hopeful parents buy techniques to select not just their child's sex but other traits as well—appearance, intelligence, and all the other makings of (according to Human Genetics Alert, an independent watchdog group based in London) "designer babies." Several women's groups and the Center for Genetics and Society drafted a joint letter asking the ASRM to maintain its original stand against PGD as a tool for "family balancing." Shortly after the publication of the article in the *Times*, the ASRM issued an official statement reaffirming its earlier conclusion.

The United States currently sets no legislative limits on the applications of sperm sorting or PGD. However, many countries, particularly in Europe, have pending legislative or regulatory prohibitions on "nonmedical" sex-selection procedures. But feminists worry that increased acceptance of sex selection in the United States will legitimize its use in South and East Asian countries, exacerbating the serious problems for women in these societies with a strong preference for sons. As an article in *Fortune* put it, "It is hard to overstate the outrage and indignation that MicroSort prompts in people who spend their lives trying to improve women's lot overseas." Disability and children's rights advocates have also expressed concern both with sex-sorting procedures and with PGD.

An estimated 25 percent of Americans say they'd like to have the opportunity to select the sex of their offspring. A study out of Cleveland State University reveals that 81 percent of women, and 94 percent of men, who say they would use sex-selection techniques would prefer their firstborn to be a boy.

While some claim this desire reinforces gender stereotypes and is based on narrow definitions of an ideal boyish boy or girly girl, certainly couples offer a range of reasons for wishing for a son over a daughter, or vice versa. Lisa Belkin, in a 2000 *New York Times* article, echoed the rationale my mother gave me for strongly desiring a daughter. Many American mothers seeking a female child, Belkin wrote, "speak of Barbies and ballet and butterfly barrettes. But they also describe the desire to rear strong young women. Some want to re-create their relationships with their own mothers; a few want to do better by their daughters than their mothers did by them. They want their sons to have sisters, so that they learn to respect women. They want their husbands to have little girls. But many of them want a daughter simply because they always thought they would have one."

I came across scores of these "just because we can, ought we?" articles while conducting a fairly narrow search on the poten-

tial health risks of ART, which reminded me that medical issues are only one concern. From the comfort of my narrow
sliver of Chicago, I had considered neither the vast social
implications of ART nor the ways in which its tools could be
used to harm, not help, women. Only that I could and therefore I ought. My limited concerns clustered around how the
medicines would affect me in the short term—whether they'd
render me a crabby, bloated, hot-flashing basket case—and
what impact the procedures would have on our insurance
premiums.

Clearly, I'm a product of my particular place and time in
history, just like my mother before me. I grew up in a demo-
cratic, capitalist country where the market drives the availability of products and procedures and where demand for ART
is so large that clinics run television ads and compete with
one another for patients, offering finance plans and other en-
ticements. It stands to reason that I'd consider such widely
available, and publicly advertised, procedures more from a
consumerist standpoint—best success rates, lowest costs, ease
of use, and friendliest staff—than from one of assumed risks. In
my mind, danger lurks in the dark shadows of back alleys, not
among those who wear makeup and cable-knit pullovers, admit their physical limitations, and triumph over them on high-
definition TV.

Of course, similar tools and techniques can be applied con-
trarily, depending on differing cultural norms and political realities. Most certainly Chinese doctors and technicians (and
party officials) squirt the same cold, blue transforming jelly
from the bottles that make a noise like squeezed mustard onto
the bellies of women just like me, only pregnant. They may
even use the same brand of ultrasound equipment that my fertility doctors and technicians rely upon to assess reproductive
possibility—the machines in China scoping out fetuses for ex-
pulsion, those in suburban Chicago divining when and if my
ovaries are filled with ripened eggs, when and if my uterine lin-

ing is ready, and when and if fertilized embryos have implanted.

I can't help but draw other similarities between the work done at rural Chinese hospitals and the offerings at fertility clinics connected to U.S. hospitals. Both have keen economic interests. Fertility treatments, costing an average of $10,000 for a single round of IVF, generate millions of dollars in income. Patients are charged for a laundry list of services: injection teaching seminars, medications, cycle management, sonograms, anesthesia. To these mandatory items, one can add other options—ICSI, cryopreservation, egg donation—to up the chances of having a baby. But at thousands of dollars per option, even the base list quickly adds up, though when physically engineering your baby, I can't imagine trying to value-engineer him or her as well.

Chinese hospitals likewise use abortion and sterilization procedures to make major *jing* from local women and visitors from neighboring Hong Kong who find it easier to travel across the border and pay about five hundred fifty Hong Kong dollars (approximately sixty-five U.S. dollars) for an abortion than to go through the formalities that Hong Kong hospitals require. (Abortions are voluntary in Hong Kong, where no family restrictions exist.) I can't help but think of those pregnant women anxiously trekking to Huaiji to void what I travel to Highland Park to try to create. Talk about your reverse commutes.

I consider myself incredibly fortunate to live in twenty-first-century Chicago and not in ancient or modern China, since I've always wanted three or four kids, and make most of them girls, please. Although from where I sit—in my car, destination Great Lakes Fertility—it is wishful thinking that I'll have any. The information I've gathered since receiving my diagnosis of Polycystic Ovarian Disorder, the hundreds of websites, TV infomercials, meetings with doctors, and fertility center seminars make clear that I shouldn't assume anything about pregnancy, neither my ability to achieve it nor my body's ability to withstand it for forty weeks.

And even if I can have a child, doing it via technology means my firstborn might very well be multiples. What then, Mom? Will I choose one—the elder, even if only by two minutes—and do all my experimenting on him? Or will I spread the guinea-pigging around? Should I nail a clipboard to the end of each crib and record how long I let this one cry it out, how that one responds to side versus back sleeping?

When my mom said "the first one is for practice," she wasn't suggesting that first children are any less important than subsequent ones. She only meant that first-time parents face a steep learning curve, and that inevitably first children suffer at rookie parents' hands: hands that hold too tightly, push too hard, compulsively flip flash cards, pile on too many layers in cold weather, or strip off too many layers in the heat.

What interests me more is how my mom took for granted that she would not only get pregnant but would do so on demand. "A year and a half between kids, at a minimum, three years at an absolute maximum," she'd advise. And instead of resenting her reproductive assumptions, instead of questioning her naïveté, I'm relieved she never had cause to doubt that I, like she, could have kids. In the late 1960s, when I was born, if you couldn't get pregnant, you either adopted or remained childless.

Even had the technology existed back then, I firmly believe that my mom, bless her artistic, expansive, nurturing heart, lacks the mettle to have undergone a successful IVF cycle, what with all the precise measuring of medications and strict scheduling. On the other hand, as an unflinchingly religious woman, she may not have been plagued, as I've been, by the nagging questions that reproductive technology stirs up. Like, if it's a doctor manipulating my system, fetching Gary's and my genetic material and combining it to produce fertilized eggs, where is God's hand? Where is natural selection? How far should we go to ensure that our investment of time, emotion, and money yields a healthy baby? If I get pregnant with multiples, do I "selectively reduce" to help assure one live, healthy birth? What is my moral responsibility to unused embryos? How will I deal with the guilt if all this tinkering with heretofore natural systems induces disease in me or, so much worse, in my children?

My mom believes unquestioningly in God, prays each morning before getting dressed, and attends temple and Torah study sessions regularly. Her religion provides a framework for how she lives her life and answers for when things go wrong. I've seen her faith in action and watched her shield herself with it when messy situations arise. Dead parents? With God. Dying sister? Almost with her parents with God.

I'm different. As much as I pray throughout the course of my day, *Please, God, make Phoebe the dog not eat so much that she barfs*, or *Thank you, God, for this awesome parking spot*, I invoke Him on nonessential issues. It's the big things, the things reproductive technology conjures, that put me in a tailspin. The questions crowded in from the get-go. First and foremost I wondered if I shouldn't just trust in nature's wisdom and leave my reproductive incapabilities alone. There was a reason I couldn't get pregnant, a medical diagnosis. So who am I to tinker with God's Plan and/or Mother Nature?

I've also considered my situation from a Praised Be He–type religious angle, wondering if I should put my faith in an all-knowing yet benevolent God who shall, at an unspecified miraculous point in the future, deliver a son or daughter unto me, patient member of His flock. Or is He a puritanical smiter, my infertility a pox upon me for my lapsed faith, my premarital sexual experience, and my all-around enjoyment of the fruit of the vine and the leaf of the plant? To that end, I wonder if I shouldn't just come to grips with my childless earthbound future and eventual eternity of hellfire and damnation.

But I desperately want pregnancy, and the fact that the science is so easily accessible, a mere matter of signing up with one of numerous area fertility clinics, makes it hard to resist even if I'm troubled that we'll spend more money to try to have a child than most people ever have to feed, house, clothe, and educate already-existing ones. And it bothers me that there are children out there who could use a loving home and that I am choosing to expend our resources in pursuit of a future one. I wish I could somehow share the technological wealth with African women who lose fetuses, and their own lives, because, in a way, they're in the modern obstetric dark.

But a force, an inner drive, is pushing me toward IVF. And anyway, if it works, we can still adopt. And anyway, there's a good chance it might not work.

4

Humanly Possible

Baby Lucy had a tinted plastic face and a heavy cloth body like a farmer's tan. Blue-plaid butterfly barrettes perched on either side of her center part, holding back hair that I wished were mine—dark, straight, and so shiny it reflected the can lights in our house. "Mama," she'd cry when tilted in any direction. "Mama," she said, as I pushed her stiff eyelashes beneath the tips of my fingernails.

For a few years I took Lucy with me everywhere, told people who would listen that I had "borned" her. On errands with my mom I'd fasten her into a car seat rigged from a toboggan pad and some rope, long before child restraints became de rigueur, when I was still sliding all over the backseat of our wagon while my brother David wedged himself upright in the front, knees locked and hyperextending, head pushing into the upholstered roof as if he were the only thing between it and a cave-in.

Those were the days of relatively carefree parenting, before the studies linking classical music to in utero possibility, back when sensory-stimulating toys consisted of pots and pans and Operation's buzzer, the red glow of its goofy-looking patient's lightbulb nose. Before all the data about what you can do to turbocharge fetal development, all this information that can make you crazy—if, say, the prenatal vitamins make you nauseous so you stop taking them, classical music puts you to sleep at work so you stop listening to it, amniocentesis is too risky so you decline. All these ways in which, even before we become parents, we're already convinced we're shitty parents.

My mom describes this as the era of voodoo gynecology, baffling terminology, patient passivity, and the paternalistic, all-knowing, all-male "female doctor." My parents were newlyweds, and my mom, dying for a baby and devastated following a miscarriage, visited her ob/gyn. Examining her uterus (tipped) and discussing her menstrual cycle (erratic), he told her she'd never bear children, what with the double whammy of abnormal uterine position and haywire periods. What she didn't know, and what he didn't explain, is that the uterus is attached to the vagina in a way that allows it to bob and weave, shift and pivot, and that a tipped uterus will in no way prevent pregnancy. A uterus, like a vagina, is potential space, hanging out in whatever position until required—to accommodate a filling bladder, for intercourse, or for pregnancy—to flex.

Believing that her doctor knew best and her body was deficient, my mom accepted her fate. She swallowed hard, shared the bad news with my dad, a few close friends, and most difficult of all her parents, who'd made clear their eagerness for grandkids. As it turned out, my mom's dad, Grandpa Barney, who ran a pharmacy in a medical building, had been hearing a lot of buzz about a gynecologist in the building. Dr. Johns was rumored to be professional and warm, confidence-inducing, yet thorough. He'd helped a few of Grandpa Barney's customers achieve pregnancy, even after they'd been told it'd be next to impossible, and besides, several of the nurses in the building had already visited him and raved. He told my mom he'd try to get her in.

Dr. Johns examined my mother and concluded that while her uterine position was slightly atypical, a bit retroverted, a touch prolapsed, it alone would prove no real impediment to achieving or sustaining a healthy pregnancy. He also taught her that she could track her menstrual cycle, irregular or not, in two ways to pinpoint her superfertile days. First, he gave her a kit containing a basal body temperature thermometer and chart and demonstrated how to use them. At the top of the graph were the days of a cycle, numbered from one to thirty-one. Before getting out of bed in the morning, she was to take her temperature either orally or vaginally. A spike indicated ovulation and the ideal time for intercourse. She was to keep charting thusly for a couple of months to provide her doctor, and more important herself, with a fertility map.

Dr. Johns also explained that he'd be tracking her vaginal discharge and that she should pay attention to it, too. This unfortunate gunk I've tried to ignore or hide from boyfriends, husbands, cleaning ladies, parents, roommates, and fellow Laundromat-goers, something to be monitored and indexed, rated and categorized. This substance is actually cervical mucus produced by estrogen in the first (follicular) phase of a monthly cycle, and bothersome as it can be, it is crucial to conception in several ways. It helps keep sperm alive for up to five days, protecting them from acidity in the vagina and creating a sort of reservoir to catch all useful ones, providing them a safe harbor before their swim up through the fallopian tubes. The point at which it most resembles raw egg whites (technically called Egg White Consistency Cervical Mucus) would be my mom's day of peak fertility.

Within six months my mom was in touch with the flux and flow of her body. She was empowered, educated, and pregnant.

Perhaps her experience and her ultimately successful outcome accounted for her certainty that I'd be successful, too. She never doubted it, at least not out loud or to me. But recognizing how much more complicated my situation and therapies were, she deems hers a primitive fertility treatment, albeit a powerful political experience. Dr. Johns had not only debunked the first doctor's doom-and-gloom prognosis, he'd given my mom the tools for taking charge of her own fertility.

To prepare for her new baby, my mother quit drinking and, based upon Dr. Johns's strong recommendation, restricted her caloric intake, lest she gain too much weight. (My mother-in-law, Bette, reports taking prescribed diet pills during pregnancy, starving herself before obstetrics appointments, and gorging on McDonald's immediately afterward, to keep from disappointing her doctor.) She picked out some baby gear without regard to the distance between slats in the crib or lead in the paint, because, she offers without hesitation, who thought about those things in the 1960s?

But mostly she spent the nine months worried about how much delivery might hurt. In those days there were no birth plans or discussions about pain management with a doctor, midwife, nurse practitioner, or doula. You labored, sans medication, until right before the actual birth, at which time the gas mask was mercifully lowered. You'd awaken in a regular hospital room, sheets and blankets tucked snug around your only slightly deflated body, and a nurse, upon request, would bring in your clean and swaddled newborn. You'd never see the mess, your partner (known as your husband back then) would never see the birth, busy as he'd be pacing, or reading the paper, in the smoky waiting room.

Now, as a precondition for delivering a baby, many obstetrical practices require expectant parents to attend a multiday prebirth seminar at the hospital with a punny, literary name like Great Expectations (although, as it turns out, The Human Stain is more apt). These long-winded marathons begin with a discussion of the stages of labor, then move on to options for pain management (a handheld showerhead aimed in the direction of the laboring mother's abdomen, a squirt of distilled water on her sweaty brow, these watery ministrations that I, for one, would clarify were not aggressive enough choices); what the laboring woman needs from her partner (photographs of the family cat waved before her to remind her of home, or perhaps to distract her with thoughts of toxoplasmosis or the accumulating hairballs that will lodge in the gullet of her newborn, or as a reminder to install guardrails around her baby's bassinet to keep Tiger clear of breath-sucking-out range); a peek into a vaginal birth, another into a cesarean section; and finally, at the end of day two, practicing one's parenting skills—diapering, nursing, burping, and swaddling—on smudged and tattered dolls you barely want to touch, let alone mock-nurse.

Those were the days when your dad let you take sips of his Glenfiddich and puffs of his smokes. Mothers encouraged their children to spend every last summer hour out in the sun, soaking it up for maximum absorption, convincing you that all the freckles you were getting were like tiny storage pods for sunlight and warmth that would release the summer slowly back into your system the rest of the cold, gray Midwestern year. Dinners centered on a chop or a strip and breakfast wasn't complete until your spoon scraped the sandbarlike heap of sugar at the cereal bowl's bottom. We had a pantry filled with toaster pastries and potato chips and no rules about when we could eat them.

I did, however, glimpse the future, a parallel existence with stringent rules and anxieties over how our lifestyles influence our health. My friend Isabelle Hollister's mother was earthy and anxious, a raw food devotee, and a believer in holistic medicine. I'd invite myself over, not only because I loved the smell of the fresh herbs her mother grew on their windowsills, but mostly because it was like visiting another planet. Their house was sort of Quakerish—unadorned floors, sparse furnishings, and wooden chairs with straight-up-and-down backs, and her mom's collection of vintage rug beaters, despite the lack of rugs, hung up on the kitchen wall. Our house, by contrast, was filled with wildly patterned wallpaper and shag carpets, velvety cushions, and framed family photographs. But the essential difference between the Hollisters and us, beyond our two ungroomed dogs and three un-litter-box-trained cats, besides my mom's Venetian-style mirrors, was the foodstuffs.

At the Hollisters' one ate not only differently, healthfully, wholly, and rawly, but at specified times. Breakfast and dinner were scheduled, and Mrs. Hollister called the kitchen staff at school to check on the weekly menu and the availability of healthful alternatives for the two bone-thin Hollister daughters. She permitted them one snack a day, after school or in midafternoon on weekends, a choice of a rice cake or plain yogurt. By contrast, our pantry was brimming with all manner of processed and sweetened treats—from sugar-encrusted cereal puffs to orange-powder-coated curlicues, we had one delicacy-filled larder and nothing perishable in sight.

I envisioned Isabelle choosing one of our snacks and sneaking it back to her house inside her violin case. She'd take her SnoBall, say, and sit with perfect spinal alignment at the kitchen table, eager to finally enjoy eating something in that kitchen. Sensing the sugar from three rooms away, Mrs. Hollister would tiptoe to the kitchen door in her boiled-wool slippers, only to see Isabelle stuffing that crumby Day-Glo orb into her mouth. "Aha!" she'd say, then take down one of the old, twisted rattan rug beaters and dare Isabelle to swallow.

The Hollisters were pale people, anemic looking, which my mom blamed on the lack of fat or fancy in their diets. A little less flaxseed and a little more frosting, she'd recommend. But say what you will, they were never sick. When the rest of the school came down with strep and mono, there were Isabelle and Greta, hauling around their violin cases and eating the lentils the kitchen ladies had been arm-twisted into preparing. These rigid Spartan ways, the whole foods and enzymatic juices that time has proven the healthier way to eat, rendering my family's tradition of beef and brownie–centered dining, our fondue nights and creamy crepe dinners, archaic at best and, perhaps, to blame for my present-day reproductive problems, the fried chicken coming home to roost.

God knows Mrs. Hollister, despite her extreme skinniness and strident ways and the undeniable fact that that lady was no sexpot, had two babies, no problem. Yet she'd tell her young girls that having grandchildren wasn't important to her, that she'd prefer for the two of them to excel in their careers, become ballerinas or violinists, to be truly fulfilled as human beings and revel in their own success, families of their own be damned. And there I was, hauling around this bulky doll while my mom reminded me in spoken and modeled ways that it was important for a woman to be a mother first and that fulfillment would follow.

"What a beautiful baby you have," people at the grocery store, the dry cleaner, the post office would remark as I struggled to hold on to an unwieldy Lucy.

"Thank you," I'd say.

"She look like her father?" the Polish produce guy would ask, noting her dark straight hair and my blonde frizz.

Driving home, I asked my mom not only how kids come to resemble their parents but whom she thought I looked like. Why did some people say it was Dad while others couldn't get over my resemblance to her? I figured resemblance was an objective thing, prima facie, and not open to interpretation.

"And Mom?" I asked. "Why does the Kimmelmans' new baby look Chinese? Why would God put a Chinese baby in an American lady's tummy?"

In these few questions, I'd given my mom several different

existential and practical topics to choose from in reply. For one, she could have taken a stab at whether God is or is not ultimately responsible for putting babies inside of other people (as if there were some celestial storehouse of eternal souls queued up for their new embodiment, with God as the ultimate yenta, playing matchmaker between old, familiar souls and these fresh, new bodies, the reincarnation parallel to Larry King's marriages). She could have presented the idea of reincarnation and explained to me that some people actually claim to remember their past lives.

If, on the other hand, she felt that procreation was random, a crapshoot in which genes, not God, account for not only the way we turn out but our very existence, I'd given her the opening to explain that, too. Or what about a discussion of sex, however rudimentary or generalized or animal-kingdom-focused? She could certainly have explained adoption, mentioning that the Kimmelmans had traveled all the way to Vietnam to find a child who needed a home and a family, a mommy and a daddy.

Instead, my mom discussed whom her kids resembled, making clear that it was her family, the Shermans, and not the Kohls. She emphasized the strength of her familial genes: the small rounded nose, high cheekbones, and swayed back. How even though her babies may have started off life looking like Kohls, she said, over time we'd all morphed into younger versions of her beloved grandmother, her father, and an uncle. "All babies resemble their fathers at birth. It's nature's way of keeping them from flying the coop," she explained, having learned this from David, who'd learned it on one of the nature programs he loved watching.

"As for why resemblance isn't always clear, different kinds of people see the world in different ways." My mom is a painter and all about how people look at things. She glanced at me in the rearview mirror, watching me topple as she swerved onto our street. David, lodged in as he was, didn't budge. "Some people zero in on eye or hair color, and based on such narrow criteria, of course they'll conclude you look like your dad. But if they look a little deeper, maybe they'll notice the slope of your cheekbones, the shape of your clavicle, the way you gesture with your hands when you tell a story and realize you are all me. I'm the observant person's progenitor."

I've parsed my physical, mental, and emotional self and figured out where to apportion credit or blame, my inheritance being both the well of good fortune from which I draw my strengths and the steaming pot of crap from which my faults originate. My strong tennis stroke, comprehension skills, and cooking ability are from the well of good fortune. My farsightedness, impatience, and off-kilter uterus putting frequent pressure on my bladder all from the pot of crap.

I valued being able to draw straight lines between the present and the past and wanted to cast that line out into the future. Someday my parents would die, I knew, and I'd be bereft when it happened, but I'd take solace in the fact that I'd extended our familial lines, given my folks yet another generation upon whom to pin their hopes, a new group of people to think about and rejoice in before breathing their last breaths. I have a hyperawareness of mortality and the impermanence and eventual inevitable disappearance of just about everything around me (except the diapers I know I shouldn't use but that absorb, fasten, stretch, and stack so perfectly), but the idea of the recurrence of certain traits, the continuance of our particular DNA structures long after we are gone, that little pinch of me that I inherited, like a sourdough starter, that my kids have and might possibly pass along—well, all that just comforts me. That is, when I'm not freaking myself out with thoughts of eternal nothingness and resenting the hell out of the Huggies that'll outlast me.

As for Gary, his undeniable and somewhat freakish resemblance to his father, Steve—height, hair, chin, vocal timbre and inflection, pronouncing a *g* at the end of a word as a *k*—is a thingkg of mutual pride. Gary has this kind, civic-minded, athletic, and youthful dad who is beloved in our town. The local pharmacist, he answers medical questions gratis and opens his store each Halloween to all costumed comers to take whatever candy bar they like, it's on him, Happy Halloween.

Every now and again Gary will notice somebody watching him. His first thought will go to food in his teeth, oil spots on his shirt, a gaping fly. But what usually follows—unless it's me or his mom studying him, in which case his first assumption is bound to be correct, unless his hair needs cutting—is "You must belong to Steve Feinerman." This comforting idea lends Gary a sense of belonging not available to us chameleons who resemble both or neither of our parents, or who never laid eyes on both or either of our parents.

When Steve dies—a fate that'll probably befall him before it does Bette, due not only to statistical norms but to Bette's fanatical diet and exercise schedule—I imagine she will want to be around Gary nonstop, an extension of the husband she has lost. *Call me Bette, not Mom,* she'll insist. *Call me during the day and ask me what's for dinner. I'm begging you.* Or maybe it'll go completely the other way. She'll refuse to see us, make up excuses as to why she doesn't want to come over for Chinese on Sundays anymore.

Gary is scads worldlier than his parents: he eats curry, uses Tabasco, trekked around Turkey. Steve fears flying over bodies of water, so he won't leave North America, and Bette distrusts the highway, so she won't leave her subscribed area without an escort. And despite his looks and his voice, Gary is an essentially different kind of person from his parents—proof to me, by negative implication, that adopted kids can share traits, or not, with their adoptive parents, proof that biology need not always be destiny, proof that connectedness between parent and child is a many-faceted and mostly intangible thing. Be that as it may, both Gary and I felt strongly that, if humanly possible, we wanted our kids to be our blood relatives.

Unquestionably we would do whatever it took to have kids that looked, smelled, and seemed like us. In the first, most practical place, we had primo health insurance; it was Illinois-based and therefore, by state law, covered four full cycles of IVF. Not using it, we figured, would be like skipping courses during a prix fixe meal, and we, for one, do not like to waste food. We also lived in a metropolitan area with ART clinics galore. We'd do our homework, shopping for the right clinic like we would any other commodity. We'd interview the doctors, nurses, and willing patients. We'd examine the wall of baby pictures, this ubiquitous display in all fertility clinics, like the plastic food dioramas in Japanese restaurants, to judge for ourselves how cute, robust, and normal their goods.

Even more than that, I had a mounting irrational desire to be pregnant. I had taken seriously the line spoken by the rabbi who had married us: "May you grow into thousands of myriads." Those words underscore one of the primary purposes of Jewish marriage, to have children who will have children, down through the generations, with me not only as the mother of myriads but as the child of them, too. This placed pressure on me not to be the point at which my grandparents' lines died, a generational black hole.

I'd watched friends and family members take their pregnancies for granted, going skiing and Rollerblading in defiance of their doctor's warnings, eating feta and blue cheese and saying they really shouldn't but couldn't resist. I'd be the perfect gestating station, committing myself to exercises, Kegel and aerobic. I'd eat healthfully and master the proper installation of a car safety seat by poring through the enclosed literature, studying the diagrams, affixing all straps and buckles, even the optional ones, registering it with the manufacturer in case of a product recall, and dropping by the local firehouse for a second, expert opinion.

We know plenty of people who went to extremes to bear their own biological children. We know others who chose adoption, either domestic or from far-flung locales. So what's the difference between these folks? Some who adopted were single parents lacking the stamina, desire, or resources for assisted reproduction. Others didn't want to become pregnant or feared passing on a genetic disorder. Still others were physically unable to have children, a fact they realized only after several failed attempts at ART.

A surprising number of our friends admit that they dreaded the thought of perpetuating familial traits. They cop to not-so-terrific gene sets, replete with cruel grandmothers, neurotic siblings, obsessive-compulsive fathers, and chronically ill mothers. They concluded that the only responsible action, as far as both they and the world were concerned, was to use their obvious good judgment to raise unbiologically related children.

Becca and Mitch, friends of ours, began trying to conceive within the first few days of their marriage (a kinky twist on their already adventurous sex life). They tried for a year to get pregnant and, failing that, ended up turning to a fertility doctor. The doctor put them through the usual battery of tests and discovered a microdeletion on Mitch's Y chromosome, a genetic trait that often results in azoospermia, or the total absence of sperm in the semen. Mitch, being completely secure in his masculinity and one of those Zen souls willing to take life as it comes, cared not at all if Becca proceeded with another man's seed as her reproductive lifeblood. When the doctor offered to try to retrieve even a couple of sperm from his epididymis to be used in IVF—that'd be all ICSI would require—Mitch declined. He worried that if it worked, if Becca got pregnant and they ended up with a son, that child would carry the same Y chromosome microdeletion, passing on the infertility that should have been nipped in the bud. When their fertility doctor suggested they use techniques to conceive a daughter, Mitch and Becca demurred, discomfited by the extra manipulation these efforts would require.

They decided on intrauterine insemination (IUI) using donor sperm. Eight cycles later Becca still wasn't pregnant, but she was disgusted. She felt bad, physically and spiritually. She had also developed a deep animosity toward the fertility clinic nurses, those "callous robots" who acted surprised by her frustration. "You only just got started," they'd say, reminding her that it routinely took years to get pregnant and assuming that she and all of their patients were aware of and resigned to this fact.

"I didn't want to spend three years trying to get pregnant," Becca says. "I just wanted to be a mom."

After that eighth attempt Becca and Mitch decided to throw in the genetic towel. Since they had already confronted letting go of 50 percent of a biological relationship, accepting that their child would have a stranger's characteristics to some degree, it was fairly easy for them to let go of it all.

"Once I knew I wasn't having my husband's babies," Becca says, "I just wasn't that excited about having my own. I wasn't. His family is so normal, and mine is so not normal. I was counting on athletic kids with all his good qualities."

Rather than order more sperm and pray that the specimen would be strong enough to eclipse Becca's family stock, they closed their account at the sperm bank and threw away the last of the liquid-nitrogen dry shipper tanks. Instead they started putting together a scrapbook, a sort of two-dimensional beauty pageant to convince a birth mother that they were the right people for her to turn her baby over to. Over time they ended up adopting two children and, as Becca says, can't wait until it's time for them to head off to college.

Among our other friends and acquaintances who decided against ART, some lacked the health insurance they needed to afford the treatment. Others, in which only one of them, due to either health or gender, would be biologically related to the child, decided that that dynamic would be too emotionally complicated. Finally, we knew plenty of people who witnessed the strains ART can place on a relationship and decided it wasn't worth the risk.

Some of our friends clung to IVF for dear life out of some sense of ethnic obligation, religious expectations, or a husband they worried might leave them if they couldn't deliver a baby. But so many others adopted children right off the bat, or served as foster parents, or decided their lives wouldn't end if they didn't have kids at all.

But are there essential differences between us? Do people with a Welsh ancestry carry an adoption impulse, while Germans favor ART? Is a left-brained gal more likely than a right-brained one to seek out technological treatments? Beyond issues of affordability and access, how can some people resign themselves so easily to one option or the other?

If my particular makeup provides an answer, people with Russian heritages, weaknesses in math, and tendencies toward nonsequential thought patterns will choose ART every time. Green Bay Packers fans and critics of those preachy yellow point-of-purchase Support Our Troops magnets will go to technological extremes for their own biological children. But that's not to say I didn't seriously reflect on other options as well. I imagined our life without children, concluding we'd end up divorced, following several years of alienation caused by an unspoken but palpable resentment. I also considered adoption, knowing that if ART ended up not working, it would be the thing I'd push for. But I was eager to try IVF first and shared these thoughts with Gary.

Playing devil's advocate, he listed the benefits of adoption and reminded me how little we still knew about the effects of reproductive drugs on a woman's system. He also brought up my anxiety about the human impact on the environment.

"If we adopted kids, we would reduce, reuse, and recycle by placing an already extant person," Gary said.

"I thought you really wanted to try to have our own kids. Biologically ours, I mean," I said.

"I do. I just want you to consider all the options, the potential harms, and how difficult this might be. What happens if IVF doesn't work? You're not going to blame me for not warning you, right?"

"I promise. Trust me. I'm thinking hard about it, considering every possible scenario, and I just know that this is the right thing for me. For us. I grew up thinking I'd get pregnant, never mind the fact I didn't really understand how that worked. Nor could I have imagined our present state of affairs. I dreamed that one day I'd be in a birthing room, and a doctor would be yelling at me to push, push! And I'd feel this sudden sense of relief as the baby finally came out, and then the doctor would be suctioning stuff out of the baby's mouth or nose or wherever, and then he'd hold the baby up, Kunta Kinte style, and I'd lay eyes on her for the first time, and then when she graduated from Harvard, I'd think back to those first few moments of our life together and get this huge lump in my throat, and she'd scan the crowd for me and, finding me, wave and give the thumbs-up."

"First of all," Gary said, "she's going to Yale. Second, it would be our baby, and she'd look for both of us in the crowd. At the Yale, not the Harvard, graduation."

Katie, a woman I know with two adopted sons, thinks kids are kids and that, more important, all parents are alike in an essential way. As she puts it, wanting to have kids, be they biologically related or not, is a purely selfish feeling on the would-be parent's part. And she's right: What do kids who don't exist know from being alive? Imagining all the couplings that had to take place for us even to exist, the happenstances and chance meetings, the persistent great-great-grandfathers, back through time immemorial, who refused to take *no, nyet, nee, nein,* or *non* for an answer, convinces the existential among us that our being here is not only a complete crapshoot but somebody else's doing.

The reincarnationists, the religious, and the fatalists may argue. But take just one body part—your wrist, say—and really check it out. It's bony on one or both sides, thick or thin, veiny or wrinkly or a particular hue—not because you are Thomas Aquinas reincarnate and he had especially delicate wrists and henceforth so unto you; and not because God created you in His image, and by looking at your wrist, you also gaze upon the spot God would wear his watch if He weren't all-knowing. Rather, your wrist is the way it is because of the specific physical histories of the thousands of generations of people over the hundreds of thousands of years that they coupled up, bore, and raised all your modern Homo sapiens ancestors—your mammoth-hunting grandmas and your wheel-getting-used-to granddads, your bubonic plague–suffering grandmothers and those Ptolemy-dissing grandfathers, all the way up to the present, to the grandparents and parents now wishing they'd see you more often or telling you what they really think of Clinton and Bush, Imus and Lohan.

What motivated early Homo sapiens to have children, I'd guess, is roughly the same thing that motivates us today—the biological desire to pass along our genetic material, to receive reflected glory, to experience vicarious joy, and to have built-in caregivers for our dotage. When folks, Cro-Magnon or postmodern, decide to have kids, it's because they're convinced they are good-parent material, or that their child will be adorable, which will reflect well on them as the source of all those good-looking genes. When the kid excels in school, people will associate the parental brain with the child's. When the kid quarterbacks the football team or stars in the school play or wins on *American Idol*, it'll all be because of you—your genes, your influence, your impeccably skillful parenting. You, that's who.

Several of our gay friends talk about increasing numbers of babies in their formerly hip, adultcentric neighborhoods. They call these children, the sons and daughters of their same-sex-coupled friends, "gaybies." They point to several phenomena around these children, the fact so many of them have old-fashioned names: Gus and Ruby, Sam and Myrtle. They also observe—somewhat unscientifically, but it's fascinating nevertheless—that lesbians tend to be more interested in adoption than male couples, and that the people they know going to extremes to have their own, genetically related progeny are almost always men.

This seemed counterintuitive. After all, it's the female of the species who's desperate for pregnancy, right? We're the ones who romanticize motherhood and babies, even in their earliest stages. We imagine how we'll react when discovering we're pregnant, we fantasize about our developing fetuses, studying ultrasound images and imagining how our worldly actions, the music we listen to, the tones of our voices, the foods we eat, will reverberate in utero. Weightless and still, even as we lumber about and negotiate life, our developing babies connect us to our basic selves. We plan for our deliveries, launder tiny outfits, and sterilize our homes. We're the ones who, as girls, happily play with faux-defecating Baby Alive dolls, mixing up the diarrhealike food to be fed to, and wiped from, these girlhood amusements.

Reproduction is so much more complex for male couples, since at a minimum, it requires three basic factors—sperm, egg, uterus—and men can't lay claim even to a majority. So what gives? Perhaps it's because male couples have higher disposable incomes and can afford ART; perhaps this is an issue neither of biology nor of instinct but of class. Certainly, the historical difference between men's and women's incomes has resulted in part in the present-day income gap between gay male and lesbian couples.

Still, the need for eggs and a gestational surrogate makes ART a particularly expensive option for gay men. A gestational surrogate can cost tens of thousands of dollars. Egg donation costs around $20,000 on average, and if you factor in the cost of in vitro fertilization of the egg, the investment is huge, an unavoidably complicated undertaking. Some gay male friends of ours did IVF using one partner's sister's eggs, the other partner's sperm, and a gestational surrogate in California, and they had a daughter. Two years later, when they wanted another child, they switched it up, using the partner's sperm, the other partner's sister's egg, and the same surrogate. Success again.

Another gay male couple used a gestational surrogate for their three children. They entrusted the surrogate with nourishing their developing fetuses and watched her give birth to their first two daughters. During an ultrasound, while she was pregnant with their third child, she asked if they'd be willing to donate sperm to her and her partner. (They were a lesbian couple.) Our friends didn't feel comfortable having only half–biologically related kids who lived not in Miami but in Oregon and whose mothers weren't interested in including the sperm donors in the children's day-to-day lives. But as the request came during the surrogate's third trimester, and they were somewhat over a barrel, they agreed.

Meanwhile, Gary disagrees with my assumption that the female of the species has the stronger reproductive drive. "We men have a biological need to spread our seed," he says. "Do you really think we'd get married if we didn't? No offense, hon."

Sometimes adopting a child truly alters the course of his or her life, saves it outright, or offers enhanced opportunity and a future. These instances transcend either biological imperative or the primary desire to fill an empty vessel with all your goodness, or repair a cracked one with your brand of glue. But the oft-made assumption that any adopted child is a saved child, that all adoptive parents are saints or miracle workers, the Mother Teresa at the PTA, is reductive and, according to several friends and professionals in the adoption community, often based on racism, classism, or elitism.

Our friends Patsy and Meg, who adopted Michael at just under three years old from a Russian orphanage, bristle at the assumption, and the intended praise they get over and again, that they saved his life. *You must feel so good about what you did,* they hear. *You guys are lifesavers,* as if they were rescuers rather than the slightly clueless, wannabe moms that they were, as if they knew all along that this Michael even existed and that he was waiting for the two of them and the two of them only. The truth is, they'd intended to go to China and bring home a little girl. They had so many friends who had done the same and assumed it would be no problem. They signed on with an international adoption agency with a ton of experience in China, filled out every last paper, shined at their interviews, and were approved.

But then the 2000 Olympics happened. During the broadcast a John Hancock Financial Services advertisement unrolled before couchfuls of Americans. The ad shows two women in line at a crowded immigration office. They're ogling a beatific Asian infant sleeping in the arms of one of them. "Hi baby, this is your new home," one whispers. Glancing around the chaotic office, the other woman jokes, "Don't tell her that. She's going to want to go back." "Do you have her papers?" It's now clear they are a couple. "Yeah, they're in the diaper bag." They smile at this. A diaper bag, a notion so domestic as to tickle them. "The diaper bag. Can you believe this? We're a family." The tagline appears: *Insurance for the unexpected. Investments for the opportunities. John Hancock.* The visuals cut out, but the audio continues. "You're going to make a great mom," one woman says. Her partner replies, "So are you."

Soon afterward Patsy and Meg were gearing up to head over to meet some babies, when the Chinese adoption door closed to anyone indicating on an adoption application that they were a single parent—a common cover for same-sex couples who know better than to categorize themselves as such. Since the agency they'd contracted with also placed Russian children, and since Patsy and Meg freely admit that they don't readily do infants of any species (when looking to adopt a dog, they fixed ten months as their minimum age), an almost-three-year-old suited them just fine. They liked the fact that by the time they took the child home, they'd already have a good sense about whether or not he had fetal alcohol syndrome, autism, or any other problem that crops up in infancy. He'd be more of a known quantity, health-wise.

As to whether they made Michael's life any easier, they're honest in acknowledging that he most likely traded in one set of problems for another, deeply complicated one. He has two mommies, and even though studies conclude that children of gay and lesbian parents show no differences from those raised by heterosexual ones, poor Michael has two moms loving him to pieces. Yes, he gets twice the cuddling and nurturing and unconditional love, but he also has two deeply dedicated people directing their laser foci on his manners and posture. They demand he respect his surroundings and liberties, their multitudinous pets, other children and teachers, authority figures, and women. All these lessons that one mother normally crams down a son's throat lovingly served up in helping after helping.

Meg, Patsy, and I share a concern about how our kids' beginnings affect them in the present. They don't know much about what may or may not have occurred during the nine months Michael spent in an unknown and untraceable mother's womb (she left a false name and address at the hospital) or during the nearly three years he spent in the orphanage. Even so, several of the children from the same facility ended up in Chicago with families who are committed to monthly get-togethers. He seems happy to see these children, his surrogate siblings, but their common experiences in Russia don't come up. They're too busy running around, eating pizza, and guffawing at American cartoons.

Sure, Michael has genetic potentials that Patsy and Meg will never know about, unless a problem arises, and even then, who's to say for sure? They puzzle over Michael's behavior, especially the fact that in his first year in this country he distinguished himself as the nucleus of most fights at his school. Was its cause hereditary, a tempestuous genetic stock? Or had Michael been bullied in the orphanage? Was he manifesting deep feelings of abandonment? Was he simply angry at being involuntarily moved across the world to this foreign house, with all its handcrafts, dogs, cats, and birds? Or was it just typical little-boy stuff?

I look at my kids and have to wonder if their behavior— good, bad or otherwise—is the result of nature, nurture, or something extra, a new factor that ART introduced. When Anna throws a fit over my inability to decipher her typically toddler-muddled enunciation (*Eedirt?* What the hell is *Eedirt?*) or Lily clings to me for dear life in the company of strangers, I question whether it's genetic, environmental, or perhaps technological. The relentless engineering that my pregnancies required had to leave some mark, I figure. From the egg cultivation and nabbing to the sperm culling and injecting, the first few days these developing clusters spent, not in a warm, supple uterus but in a rigid, artificially lit petri dish, these precarious cleavage-stage embryos doing their crucial cell division, not where God or nature intended but in a man-made embryo medium culture. Subsequently we examined, judged, and selected the embryos and transferred them into the uterus by means of a catheter, all of these ways in which we manipulated Sophia's, Anna's, and Lily's lives before they were even officially around.

5

Professionals

Carol, Great Lakes Fertility's head nurse, is universally regarded by the patient population as one tough mother. Uninterested in individual circumstances and intolerant of emotional displays—a box of generic tissue paper positioned at her desk's edge is the only hint she recognizes any potential for tears or snot, whether generated by anxiety or sorrow, allergies or the common cold—Carol goes about her business as if it were any ordinary business, as if she were selling insurance or hocking used cars. "I hate her," women in the waiting room gripe to their husbands or fellow patients, who nod and say, "Me too, me too."

Stories of her iciness circulate around the waiting room, a whispered refrain uniting us rebuffed. One report had Carol shushing a weeping patient with a nearly ten-second shush. Its volume rising toward its climax, making the crier cry even louder, at which point Carol reportedly commanded, "Can it. People are trying to work back here." I myself have heard her censure lively coworkers with variations on this packaging theme—canning, putting corks in or lids on, these homespun admonishments to keep one's shit together or the whole place could blow. As part of our intake, Carol reminded each and every one of us (rumor had it) that we were neither the first to go through these procedures nor Great Lakes Fertility's only patient. We needed to be tolerant and courteous and mindful not to take our personal frustrations or hormonal shifts out on the staff members, who were doing their best to speed us through our appointments as quickly and effectively as possible. She implored us to identify a partner, friend, or confidante with whom we could share our frustrations, since the staff would prove rather terrible hand-holders, that's how busy they were, that's how many hands needed holding.

I tried putting myself in Carol's shoes (pastel orange nurse numbers). What kind of misanthrope would I be if my job required me to deal daily, weekends too, not only with hundreds of people hankering for babies, but with the truly desperate ones, insecure and pushy dudes forced into confrontations with their masculinity and bloated, destabilized women, their systems coursing with painfully injected hormones? Could I feign interest in an umpteenth tale of false fertility starts, unsympathetic partners, and deep feelings of physical betrayal? Would I make eye contact, nod my head, and murmur, *I understand, I know how hard this can be,* allowing my professional self some softness around the edges? Or were the demands placed on assisted reproductive technicians, to keep vigilant watch over scores of patients' medical regimens, taxing enough without also requiring keen people skills?

I understand. I get the detachment and the tendency toward efficiency over hospitality. It would take a saint to deal with all the technical and emotional demands. Sure, Dr. Hamlin seems to take it all in stride. But his position is easier, separate as he is from the administrative bit. He is our hero, a messiah of sorts, and we know better than to distract him from the end-game. Blood tests and scans and schedules, phone calls with exam results, and answers to our prosaic questions — *What time of the day should I administer my shots? When reconstituting the medicine, should I use distilled or filtered water? Should I clean the site with alcohol before and after the shot, or just before? Should I let the alcohol evaporate completely before inserting the needle? Which thigh, the left or the right?* — are for the nurses and lab techs to process, with Carol as helmsman. So of course she is crabby, physically and mentally present as she has to be for early-morning blood tests, evening ultrasounds, and all the hours in between.

Not that we patients aren't peevish. In fact, many of us are downright depressed. According to the Mind/Body Medical Institute, a nonprofit scientific and educational organization that studies mind-body interactions and their medical application, infertility can cause insomnia, fatigue, physical pain, and hostility. Looking around Hamlin's waiting room, at the pasty and the miserable, the baggy-eyed and the irritable, I decide that that is some spot-on conclusion. In addition, research confirms that infertile women are twice as likely to have depressive symptoms as are fertile women, a particularly damning finding since depression contributes to infertility, causing one to question which comes first: the down-in-the-dumps chicken or its empty nest. Studies show that women experiencing infertility are as depressed as women with AIDS, HIV, and cancer, and that depressed women who undergo IVF are only half as likely to conceive as nondepressed women. The more depressed we get, the more we retreat from social interactions, avoiding not just our normal activities but our friends and family, particularly those with babies, since, the truth is, we're utterly jealous, and the more ashamed of ourselves we feel, the more depressed we get.

Alice Domar, Ph.D., director of the Mind/Body Center for Women's Health at Boston IVF, has written: "Procreation is the strongest instinct in the animal kingdom: males of virtually every species are willing to kill or be killed just for the chance to mate. And females of almost every species are willing to die to protect their young." This instinct naturally bleeds over into our clinical encounters. It's hard to sit tight, quietly, patiently, when the hundreds of thousands of years of human instinct stored up in your tissues are urging you to act otherwise, to put down the inane magazine, rise up, and attack! Kill the receptionist positioned between you and your genetic material! Strangle the scheduler who won't reunite you with your fertilized embryos until the third Thursday in November!

So if your A Plan, mating with the partner you selected in large part for the superior reproductive vibe he transmitted, fails and you end up in a clinic, instituting a plan that was nowhere near the top of your options list, you're going to have to stow your instincts. You hope the situation will be temporary, that once you're pregnant, you'll be able to reintegrate nature, oozing it from your swollen breasts to your fleshy ass, your glowing face to your beef-craving belly.

But for now the facts of your condition and the clinic's rules force you to act civilized, wait patiently, and turn a deaf ear to the profound questions—*What am I doing here? Where's that virile stud I married?*—circulating in your confused brain. You wonder not just about the medicine and procedures—*What are the side effects? Will it hurt? How naked will I have to get?*—but their application and whether the staff properly values your particular case. The nurses, techs, and doctors seem too casual for such grave matters, too uniformly detached in their dealings. And then you are back in that waiting room, quieting the freaking-out woman next to you who was given somebody else's medication schedule, which fucked up her cycle and possibly her system. And you try to comfort her and convince yourself that although this mistake is catastrophic, there is a first time for everything, and better her than you.

"They should have stacks of customer satisfaction surveys all around this place," a fellow patient says to me after we've been informed that only one lab technician has shown up that morning, and since he is doing all of the blood draws, it'll take twice as long. "If they do it at Denny's, don't you think they should do it here? As a PR move, at the very least. I mean, half of my problem is that nobody seems to care how I'm doing, beyond my follicular development."

I was trying to stay above the waiting-room fray, distance myself from the kvetching. (I wanted good karma and a positive attitude, but more important I wasn't convinced Carol hadn't planted bugs.) But customer satisfaction surveying was a good idea, and I told her I thought so.

"But you can be the one to suggest it," I say. "I wouldn't dare."

I decided fairly early on to put aside my assumptions, about my reproductive system, sex life, human creation, and Great Lakes Fertility's way of running their clinic. I'd squint a little and view the coming months, or years, through myopic eyes, or go insane. Look how busy they are, I'd remind myself. Check out their great success rates. The ASRM has found a strong correlation between busyness, as in attempted cycles, and improved outcomes, making this beehive a good bet. Also, the clinic was founded over twenty years ago. That's a lifetime in ART terms, considering it has been available in this country only since the late 1970s.

Louise Brown, "The Baby of the Century," was born in 1978 at Oldham General Hospital in England. That same year Benjamin Brackett, a member of the Biomedical and Health Sciences Institute and a professor of veterinary medicine, created at least one hundred healthy IVF rabbits. He commented to a *Washington Post* reporter, "We really don't know the effect of the mechanical and chemical manipulation of an egg prior to fertilization," but the stats since 1978 have been reassuring.

The legions of IVF babies who have turned into children, teens, and then adults appear to be normal, and the number of IVF procedures performed and their success rates have increased dramatically. In 2004, the Centers for Disease Control (CDC) reported that the rate of cycles resulting in live births was 29 percent. Some ART centers report rates as high as 50 percent live births per retrieval. The CDC places the odds of conception at between 24 and 29.5 percent per cycle, similar to the 20 to 25 percent chance that a healthy, reproductively normal couple has of achieving pregnancy that results in a live-born infant in any given month.

When Gary and I initially met with Dr. Hamlin, he assured us that with Gary's decent sperm count (despite a bit of sluggishness and slightly decreased volume in the sperm sample) and my young age, he was confident we'd conceive. "Our success rates are slightly higher than the national norm," he said. "And in the most important category—live birth rate per cycle initiated—we lead the pack." When Dr. Hamlin referred to me as young, he clarified, he meant in IVF terms rather than the biologically ideal reproductive age, which most doctors agree is a woman's twenties.

I kept the stats in mind, the quantitative and qualitative measures assuring me that I was in good hands as far as a live birth was concerned. I assumed my role as patient and understood that I'd need to suppress my most basic and strongest instincts and play nice. In fact, I'd play masterfully, not only following the rules and procedures to a T and ending up pregnant with the preferred singleton, but doing so in a way that would win Carol over. She'd be the one to phone me with the great news. And then, over the next nine months, she'd check in occasionally to say they missed me around the office and ask how the pregnancy was going: Was I tired? Was I showing? And when I had the baby, I'd send her an announcement and picture, and perhaps she'd send a small gift.

It would be like motherhood boot camp. When Carol acted surly, I'd soothe. If she seemed particularly tetchy, I'd nurture. I'd keep my cool and blame her misbehavior on factors beyond her control—hunger or fatigue or irritable bowels—and once I became a mom, I'd look back on this time as having contributed in crucial ways to my fantastic mothering skills.

I've always had an instinct for swaying acerbic coots and petulant biddies, convinced I can befriend even the foulest-mooded person. When people waiting in line at the grocery checkout would grumble about the mealy apples or the detached cashiers, I'd make eye contact, nod my head, and murmur, "I understand, I know how hard this can be," even if the produce and employees were shiny and crisp, quick and able. At least Carol was youngish, so I wouldn't have to span the chasm of age. And I really did understand her plight, though she could use some tweaking, personality-wise.

If I witnessed Carol roll her eyes at a patient or coworker, I'd smile, but only vaguely, not so much that she'd think I was laughing at or patronizing her, just enough to let her know I was simpatico. I'd offer no offense in my person, shunning perfumed lotions and loudly patterned clothes. Having already discovered the mistake of wearing running shoes with their treaded rubber soles on the clinic's highly polished floors (the resulting sound like ten thousand crickets), I'd pick quiet shoes, moccasins, or a pair of slippers that I'd keep in my bag. I'd turn off my cell phone and remove the car key from its jangly chain. I'd sit still, mummylike, and let her do all the talking.

If Carol still lashed out at me, I'd channel beekeepers and pit bull owners, Siegfried and Roy. I'd remain perfectly calm and avert my gaze—or blame myself for the resultant mauling.

———

Carol uses a clogged foot to wedge open the door separating the packed waiting room from the exam rooms and labs. "Elizabeth," she says, as if clearing her throat. At least twenty of us wait. I'm not sure she means me. I glance around to see if anyone else is moving.

"Elizabeth Westerbrook?" a blonde woman says, lowering an issue of *Ski*, "The Magazine of the Ski Life."

"I'm Meredith," the person next to me offers. "Did she say Meredith? You listen so hard for your name, but then when it's called, you're not really sure . . ."

Carol had already retreated. I rise and feel forty eyes upon me as I inch open the swinging door. Carol stands there, talking with a nurse in a medical smock covered with gardening rabbits. Rabbits pushing wheelbarrows. Rabbits dropping pawfuls of seed in straight rows. "You can't come back here until we call you," she says, noticing me.

"I'm Elizabeth Kohl Feinerman. You called 'Elizabeth,' but we weren't sure which you meant."

She checks the file she is holding. "Did you say Kohl? Or Feinerman? Because I don't have any Kohls. Just Feinerman. So if you are Feinerman, follow me. Yeah? Okay, but please don't come back here without first being called. I know I did call you, but then you came by yourself, and that's not all right. So, you can't decide on a name?"

Gary and I had met with Carol before, once for a brief chat in a hallway and again in a conference room. This was my first time in her office, which can only be described as homey. A quilt made out of old T-shirt parts hangs on one wall, "The Des Plaines Bandits" printed in the middle square. Framed pictures of towheaded children litter her bookshelves and credenza, especially of this one little girl at various stages of life, starting with a baby picture, lacy elastic around her forehead like Olivia Newton-John's sweatband, and culminating with a school picture, the smoky blue backdrop behind the now front-toothless child.

"Are those your kids?" I ask. "They're adorable." Fuck. Why had I talked? Where was my vague smile? Where was the mummy?

"That's my daughter, yes," she answers.

Carol isn't wearing a wedding ring. I look for a picture of a significant other but can't find one. Maybe she's a single mom: divorced, gay, or never married. Or maybe she'd been bored at work one day, back in the days before Hamlin's eminence, before the constant slam. She might have taken a liking to one of the sperm donors, or at least his looks and mannerisms, nabbed a bit of his surplus, and like a stylist capable of cutting her own hair, performed self-IUI.

Sickened by engineering so many new lives, perhaps she adopted. Like the architect who builds sleek, modernist high-rises but lives in a converted barn filled with folk art and chipped-painted cast-offs, maybe she maxed out on attempting to spark lives at work, preferring an actual, extant person for herself. At some level maybe she disapproved of ART, her hostility and intolerance for everyone around her a way to let us know that the planet would be a better place if all of us patients spent our money elsewhere. We should consider HIV/AIDS children, ditched preemies incubating at Cook County Hospital, or parentless brothers and sisters in international orphanages. What about *Wednesday's Child* on the local NBC affiliate? These slightly older foster children accompanying anchorwoman Alison Rosati on fantasy play dates, to basketball games or the aquarium, ending in a pitch by Ms. Rosati for a permanent home for these special kids. And then there were the wide-eyed, fly-bothered children in UNICEF ads. If we didn't adopt them or at least send them the money we were spending on IVF-related costs, who would?

A small basket filled with potpourri balances on top of Carol's computer. I envision dried lavender flakes getting swept up in a breeze, wafting next door into the lab, losing altitude, and alighting in somebody's genetic soup.

"Sit down," Carol says. "But don't bother taking your coat off. This'll be fast." She hands me a folder with a bright orange sticker on it. "You saw how crowded it is out there," she says. "It's always gonna be like that. We batch you guys."

"Batch?"

"Yes. Batch. Batch." *Bitch.* "Batch, as in group. Is that clearer? We put you all on birth control pills to synch up your cycles. Here's the prescription. Start them Sunday. I take it you're not currently on birth control." She pauses and looks at me. "Right? Right?"

"Yes."

"Yes you're not on birth control, or yes you are?"

"I'm not taking anything, no."

She squints and nods. "You'll stimulate for two weeks, and then we'll aspirate and transfer the following week or two, depending."

"Depending on what?" I ask.

"Read the packet I just gave you. Then if you have questions, write them down and raise them at your next appointment. You've been assigned a number. It's stuck to the front of your folder. When you sign in, call to make an appointment, or check on results, refer to yourself as number"—she reaches across the desk, warps back the folder, and reads the orange sticker—"two-oh-one-two-five. Did you bring your completed insurance forms? Stop next door and see Tina, our financial counselor, before leaving."

The schedule in my packet lays out my month: a baseline at the clinic—a blood draw and uterine ultrasound—then back to the city to Braun Drugs, an independent pharmacy with its own developing IVF niche, for two shopping bags filled with estrogen and estrogen-suppressing medication, progesterone gel, human chorionic gonadotropin and other synthetic hormones, Pergonal, Prednisone, patches, syringes, wrapped and premoistened alcohol squares, prenatal vitamins, baby aspirin for optimizing blood vessel action, and several pages of FDA warnings about potential adverse effects including, but not limited to, hot flashes, abdominal pain and bloating, edema, weight fluctuation, vaginal dryness, ovarian enlargement, headaches, multiple gestation, hyperstimulation syndrome, depression, decreased interest in sex, cancer.

According to my instructions, a nurse or lab tech would phone with the go-ahead to begin medication. The first three days, between six and ten p.m., I'd inject Lupron into my thigh to suppress estrogen production and then, after an ultrasound, begin injecting hormones into my belly during that same four-hour window. Then once every two days I'd return to Great Lakes for a blood test and a follicular growth evaluation. When the ultrasound revealed at least one follicle measuring in the fifteen-millimeter range, I'd be seen every day until most of my follicles reached nineteen to twenty-one millimeters in diameter. Oocyte retrieval would occur the next day. This was the point at which my partner would contribute his genetic material. The embryologist would examine the sample and inject the strongest sperm—those with the most regular but vigorous back-and-forth tail motion and evenly rounded heads, the same criteria I used for selecting our puppy—directly into the eggs using a microscopic needle.

That evening the embryologist would phone to let us know how many eggs had fertilized. The next day she'd update us on how many were still developing and at what rate. At this point, we would face a decision: Do we transfer a greater number (up to four if they all looked decent, between four- and eight-celled or thereabouts) at day three? Or do we wait until blastocyst occurs—on day five, when the embryo has two different cell types and a central cavity—thus transferring only those embryos we know are continuing to thrive and also, possibly, transferring fewer embryos to minimize our chances of a multiple pregnancy?

Based on our decision, I'd make my appointment. For the hour immediately following the procedure, I was to remain

supine in my personal recovery area, a curtained square containing a lounge chair for the patient, a less comfortable chair
for her partner or friend or stuff, and a storage bin for her
personal effects and clothes (since she'd wear a hospital gown
during the transfer). When the hour was up, I was to dress gin-
gerly—no tight waistbands allowed—and proceed with care to
my designated driver's vehicle, driving being verboten, much
less riding any way but reclined.

> Try and relax!!! [the instructions scream]. Your care is merely
> precautionary, a way to prevent you from blaming yourself in
> case pregnancy does not result. DO NOT worry the embryos
> will slip out of your body. Neither they, nor your uterus, is slip-
> pery!!! Think of the embryos as marshmallows suspended in
> your Jell-O mold of a uterus!! Remain on strict bed rest for
> three full days. Modify your activity, and practice complete
> pelvic rest for seven more days. Drive only if necessary, and
> be extremely defensive in your driving. Do not lift anything
> weighing over ten pounds (e.g., the average grocery bag).
> Return to Great Lakes Fertility for a blood test. Next steps:
> Plan A, continued blood and ultrasonic monitoring and
> progesterone support until week 12 in case of pregnancy, or:
> Plan B, skip one cycle to allow body to rest and reserve space
> in next available batch.

I read and reread the instructions, fearing I'll get something
wrong or forget a step. I don't know how to practice pelvic rest.
I try concentrating on the pelvic region, visualizing a shaft
of light massaging its several parts. This technique yields the
desired result's opposite. It also takes me a couple of reads
and some serious concentration to grasp how my uterus could
possibly resemble a gelatin dessert. Was it somehow Bundt
shaped, its sides rounded and rolling at regular intervals? I
think about hysterectomies, the contents of surgical pans cov-

ered in Cool Whip. Of course they meant viscosity, not shape or taste, a fact that eventually occurs to me.

I phone my local grocery store to ask how much the average bag of groceries weighs, dubious about the caution and convinced that Great Lakes Fertility is gilding the vigilance lily. The woman I speak with fixes the median weight at eight pounds but emphasizes that this is an average.

"Throw in a gallon of milk and a sixer of soda, and you've got yourself one heavy sack," she says. "We have young men to help carry bags to the car, you know."

"It's not that," I tell her. "I'm about to have a bit of surgery, and I just wondered if I'll be able to shop afterward, without hurting myself."

"You don't want to pop those stitches," she says.

"Yeah, something like that. I don't suppose the young men would be willing to come home with me to unload the bags from the car?"

"No, baby," she says. "They're not allowed in customers' vehicles. Once you leave our lot, you're on your own."

Great Lakes Fertility's system—their batches and strict instructions and meticulous scheduling—both comforted and discomfited me. The sheer volume of people going through the same procedures, these women I would see day after day, felt like teammates on good days and fellow prisoners on worse ones. We'd been stripped of the names chosen by our parents and amended, or not, over the course of our twenty or thirty or forty years and been assigned numbers in their place. It would have been easy to feel dehumanized, mechanized, but I figured the clinic was doing this to preserve patient anonymity, which is a big deal to a lot of people who go through this stuff. The numbers also helped group us by procedure and procedure date, with like numbers clustered to keep the batches straight, at least the first time through. It's an easy method for keeping track of individual patients, a way not to misplace files based on a spelling mistake or compound last names, like mine.

And if I had to be called by, and refer to myself as, a number, I liked the fact mine was so high, thinking that perhaps I was their 20,125th customer served. They'd had 20,124 other people upon whom to perfect their techniques, 20,124 guinea pigs who'd been examined and treated, impregnated or not. Or perhaps their numbering system was based on something less rational, some kind of code or mystical criteria with each particular number vibrating uniquely, like music, corresponding somehow to its patient. Number 111 assigned to the tightest-assed among us; 636, schizophrenic or just flaky; 1985, a woman donning gigantic shoulder pads or an asymmetrical hairstyle. And my number, 20125. So solid. Admittedly high, but youthful, somehow, what with all those zeroes, ones, and twos.

Other times, my early-morning posse and I seemed to be codelinquents doing time in juvie hall. We had a month's worth of scheduled hours, institutional furniture, and strict instructions not to wear certain types of clothes (e.g., those that constricted our waists). We were also told to avoid all alcohol since it could counteract the medication, a particularly difficult rule to follow since, try as I might, I struggled to muster the courage to stab myself in the stomach with a stinging-medicine-filled syringe without first loosening up. Better counteracted medicine than no medicine at all, I reasoned.

We were a group thrown together by circumstance: the dentist from Kenosha, seated next to the Bulgarian immigrant from Skokie, seated next to the perfectly coiffed and shod woman from Kenilworth. This motley crew, my batch. And as much as we tried to respect one another's privacy, not ask too many questions, or seek unoffered information, we all had our infertility in common, had one goal in sight, and hoped for one another's success. And when the cycle was over, and one of us didn't show up in two months for another try, we'd assume she'd gotten pregnant, feel happy for the mother-to-be and relieved that Hamlin got it right some of the time, but also be despondent, frustrated, and insanely bitter that that pregnant lady wasn't us.

I was discomfited, too. These were intimate issues, and body parts, I was ceding to strangers. Just as people who undergo open-heart surgery must reconcile themselves to having doctors tinker not only with their ticker but with their emotional fountainhead, and just as brain surgery patients must wrap their minds around doctors tapping into their central processing units, I was being forced not only to surrender my dream of mysterious, miraculous regeneration but also to allow a multitude of strangers access to my womanly parts. Like an usher shining his flashlight on the kids making out in the balcony, Dr. Hamlin would open the speculum and position the lights, and there'd go romance and earthiness and human sexual reality, laid bare and elbowed aside by an administrative one. And that was okay. I wanted to get pregnant, and I had chosen this method, this doctor. Only, with so few mysteries in life, I mourned this one's loss.

I was cool with no Kate Bush, no scratchy stubble on my face, no fingertips in the small of my back—but did there have to be so many lights? So many instruction sheets printed on colored paper? For what? To make them more festive? I understood all the appointments and monitoring, the precise directions, but having the whole thing spelled out and explained, my womanly system so easily predicted and manipulated, forced a shift in perspective. None of us is as unique or mysterious as we'd like to believe, a fact that most medical students, and whores, must realize, but that threw me for a loop.

Once I'd made the shift, resigned myself to the fact that I possessed the same body parts as most female human beings, mine being neither lovelier nor more powerful than the next, I felt better, more relaxed. Hey, it was their very commonness, their misfiring along a fairly well-worn trajectory, that enabled me to take part in the science. Hallelujah! Praise homogeneity!

I began to marvel at the brilliance of the technique and gave greater credit to these pioneers—the doctors and nurses, the embryologists and ultrasonographers. They were innovators, miracle workers. They had improved upon nature by giving otherwise infertile people the wherewithal to have children, and God bless them, my future was in their hands.

The ultrasonographer is a sports freak named George. An AM sports talk station, all male voices, mostly South Chicago accents, airs debates over athletic minutiae as George bounces ultrasonic waves off uteri. As I walk into the darkened scan lab, animated callers argue over whether Sacramento or San Antonio will win it all that year.

"Sac?" George shouts at Paulie from Bolingbrook as I slip off my pants and slide onto the table. "Is he out of his freakin' gourd? Does he actually think Vlade Divac's any match for Tim Duncan?"

"Ready," I say after smoothing the protective plasticized paper sheet down over my hips. George swivels on his stool to face the monitor.

Some ultrasonographers ask you to guide the tip of the probe into your own body. Others, like George, do it themselves. If you reach down to navigate when you're with the latter type, they act all huffy and offended.

"I hate it when cases do that," George said at my first ultrasound, when I'd instinctively reached down to put it in myself. But wasn't the other way, his way, creepy and undeniably sexual? Wasn't it meant to establish him as the dominant, technology-savvy expert and the patient, me, as the all-too-human, desperate object? Wasn't it the stuff of a fantasy (his, not mine) involving a hapless patient and her sports-maven of an ultrasound technician? "Did you take a sixty-hour certification course for this?" George asked. "Darling, I'm a pro."

He clamps the probe between his thighs, tip pointing up, and squirts blue ultrasound transforming jelly on top. He unrolls a latex condom over it and, with small strokes, unfurls it down the sides. "Are those a special type?" I ask.

"Yeah. Trojans," he says. He has gum in his mouth. Flipping up the protective sheet, he pokes around until he finds what he is looking for. "Aha! Thar she blows."

My left ovary is easily observable. Several smallish lumps the size of lima beans cluster along one wall. George uses a mouse to click on an edge of the first lump and drags an electronic line to the other side, all the while telling me who would comprise his all-time fantasy basketball team.

"The Big O." *Point. Click. Drag.* "Jabbar, of course." *Click. Drag.* "But I'm not a Bird fan. As far as honkies go, I'd choose Pistol Pete every time." I don't know how, or even if, he is tracking my follicular progress, but I want to disagree with him about Bird. Only he's jerking around inside me.

He hunts for my other ovary, which I can see off in the distance of the glowing black-and-white screen.

"You do got another ovary in there somewhere, correct?"

"Over to the right," I say, which causes him to push the wand to the left. "No. To the right," I repeat. "There. Can't you see it?"

"There it is."

"No. You already counted that one. Move to the right."

"This is the right. The tip is pointed right. See? See?" he says, pushing the thing right into my swollen, pendulous left ovary to prove his point.

"I meant pull your hand to the right."

"That's what makes me the professional, sweetie. We go by instrument, not manual, direction. Voyla. Jordan, of course, and Bill Russell. Phil Jackson would coach." *Click. Drag.*

I like what I see on the screen: great big clusters of follicles like grapes heavy on the vine, fecund and dewy. It's a sight that requires an education to appreciate. After two weeks of almost constant appointments, I know what I'm looking at, but to the novice's eyes, oddly shaped bumps that appear over the course of a few days and feed on what the body gives them must seem like textbook cancer.

I suddenly feel attached to these follicles, responsible for the fact they have made it this far and for their potential as human beings. I've seen them evolve from undifferentiated speckles to overlapping shadows to these things that I can suddenly imagine becoming complex. My eyes jump from globe to globe, trying to pick out my kid.

"Okay, sweets. You're done," George says, quickly pulling out the wand and tossing the used condom toward the trash can by the door. I watch it hit the rim and stick there. "Jump ball," he says.

"What do you think? Do they look ready?" I ask, tugging the sheet back down and waiting for George to get up and out so I can dress.

"That's not my call," he says, typing the next person's name into the machine. "That's one for my coach man, Dr. H. But between you and me, you do got some beauts."

"Really? How big?"

"Two nineteens. One or two twenties. In fact, you're probably ready to go right now. Hope by tomorrow they aren't overripe."

"Overripe? Like too mature?"

"Yep. Happens all the time. I like to think of it as a suicide squeeze. You know baseball?" he asks.

"No," I say. "Not well."

"Check it out. Your mature guys here?" He taps the monitor, which still holds the picture of my ovaries. For a moment, I worry he'll startle my embryos as if they're sleeping fish. I remind myself they are mere broadcast versions. "They're like your batter. Let's say they bunt, you know, sacrifice themselves. Some of the other guys, these little shavers here"—George

makes pinging noises to indicate which follicles he means—
"have a chance to make it home. And like any good coach, Dr.
H. only likes to use it when a patient has less than two outs."

"Outs?" I ask.

"Yeah, outs. As in, failed attempts at pregnancy. You only get
so many tries, you know. Same as baseball. Same as life."

As the month wore on and my visits to George's darkened
room added up, I became confused and found it increasingly
difficult to keep in mind my ultimate goal of a healthy, fully
formed baby person. Getting through the appointments became a sort of end in itself. You would have thought that
his two adorable daughters' headshots, taped up all over the
place, might have helped remind me of the bigger picture, especially since George said he put them there "to give patients
something encouraging and, let's face it, pretty damn cute, to
focus on."

"The older one's too quiet to ever make it big," he'd explain
while also manipulating the ultrasound wand, while also taking and typing in measurements. "But the little one's the
whole package. Sweet looking and sharp as a tack. A natural-
born mimic. I could have done much worse."

Yeah, they were cute. But I could have done without the
photos. Putting kids to work so young felt wrong, pimpish. And
how could their own dad judge them as if they were beauty
pageant contestants? I wanted George to concentrate on his
work, on my increasingly complex innards. I had also begun
to struggle to understand how the caviar serving's worth of eggs
on the monitor could ever possibly turn into any type of child,
much less ones you make up and photograph. And what would
become of the dozens of them that didn't develop? They were
taking on a life of their own—I followed their progress and
prayed for them and hated to think they'd just disappear
one day.

I asked George if he'd mind printing out the ultrasound pictures, as a way to preserve a memory, but he told me no can do. The doc needed them, and besides, he wasn't authorized to print doubles. I wanted those images, wanted to tape them to my fridge as I'd seen my sister-in-law do with her son's ultrasound picture, his microscopic fist making its way toward his undifferentiated mouth. I thought that if I could possess them, slip them into my purse, and show them to my mother, my mother-in-law, my husband, and my manicurist, I'd have taken the first step toward motherhood. I was getting ultrasounds, just like any old pregnant woman. And the revealed images were absolutely baby-related! So, for the love of God, if you could just print them out and give them to me to have something to focus on and hold on to, George, I'd be ever so temporarily satisfied.

Then I start having this recurring dream about my labor and delivery. One of those old-fashioned nurses with the cardboard triangular hat like a pierogi stands by my side, calling me "dear" and swabbing perspiration from my face. I grunt and scream, and she tells me it's okay, everything will be just fine. Gary and a masked obstetrician are there, too, staring between my sheet-draped knees, presumably at a vagina in action. *That's the birth canal,* I hear the doctor explain to Gary, who asks whether a birth canal is anatomically distinct from the part of the vagina he's used to. *I don't understand what you're asking,* the doctor says. *One more push, honey,* Gary coaches. I give it my all, and out pops my child, a nineteen-celled cluster resembling one of Willy Wonka's Everlasting Gobstoppers. *Where will I find diapers to fit this child?* I say to Gary, who is asking the doctor if there's an umbilical cord to snip and why the baby isn't crying. *Doc,* I say, *where's her mouth? I'm starting to lactate over here.*

Aspiration

Gary clenches his jaw in the predawn light, bones knobbing beneath the blue-black, day-old makings of a beard. He's looking hot and rugged in a technical insulation jacket and the heavy-duty Gore-Tex boots I picked out for him because I'd fancied them on a slightly fey ex-boyfriend. They look even better on all six feet, two hundred pounds of Gary. His cheeks and forehead are lustrous and flushed, burnished by the predawn wind shear rushing through the ten feet of yard separating our house from the garage. This guy should be commandeering a Safari Jeep, bedding beautiful women, or rescuing people and their pets from burning buildings. Yet here he is, behind the peeling leatherette wheel of a dated Volvo, shepherding his testy wife into the hands of another man and trying to psych himself up for the ejaculation of his life.

We're on our way to Highland Park for my aspiration (in which a needle is passed through the vagina under ultrasound guidance to remove the eggs) and Gary's specimen production (the usual masturbatory thing, plus a clinic-issued receptacle and a lofty goal). He's driving cautiously, trying to avoid potholes and other bumps in the road since I'm crampy and sore, my ovaries packed with dozens of mature follicles.

Over the past few weeks I'd administered a variety of medicines, rereading the directions each time to assure I was neither skipping steps nor adding new ones. Some were agents to shut off the hormones I naturally produced; others were replacement hormones; all were compactly packaged in shiny cardboard containers like miniature bento boxes. My kit had slots for the thimble-size glass bottles containing the drugs, and other, larger compartments for the tear-apart chains of premoistened alcohol towelettes and slim syringes with orange caps. Per Hamlin's directions, I'd been taking baby aspirin to amp up my vascular system and prenatal vitamins bursting with extreme amounts of folic acid to stave off birth defects in the fetus that I prayed would start taking shape in the next couple of days.

I stored the supplies in a kitchen cabinet and, when alone, would administer the drugs. I'd imagine myself a doctor or junkie, popping the tops off tear-shaped vials, peeling the crinkly tin tops off others, uncapping syringes, and expertly, or so I pretended, withdrawing 10ccs of this or that and injecting them into my thighs and my belly. I'd done a decent job of it. The last few ultrasounds revealed them, wall-to-ovarian-wall of black blobs, like the surface of the moon or an overly sausaged pizza.

Gary scratches his face, raking at his cheek as if he's trying to pick food out from the molars beneath the skin, vein, and muscle. I want to ignore it, knowing this is Gary's version of thumb-sucking, but the percussive sound of his nerves is grating, and I'm on edge as it is.

"You okay?" I ask, cueing him to knock it off.

"Fine," he says. "Why?"

"You're scratching your face in that nervous way, and it's bugging the hell out of me."

"Jeez. Sorry," he says, pausing. "You know, it's not like I don't have reason to be bothered, too."

"Oh, so now you understand how I've been feeling?" I listen to myself, not liking at all the way I sound, like a fishwife, a nag, a harpy. I can't stop. "Before you attempt an answer, keep in mind that not once in the past month have I had the great good pleasure of an orgasm—at an office or at home or anywhere else. Nor have I been the one to touch myself, despite the fact I wouldn't want to go near this current mess of a body."

"Jeez," Gary says again, looking at me, "I said I was fine. You don't have to act like such a bitch." He clenches the steering wheel, steeling himself for the fight he assumes will follow his calling me this second-most-prohibited of names. I remain silent, reassessing whether I really want to have kids with this name-calling douchebag.

To Gary's credit, until recently he'd done a fairly decent job of trying to understand my worries and the drudgery of my days. Walking in from work, he'd give my shoulder a little squeeze and ask, "How's it going today, hon?" even before heading to the fridge or loosening his tie. At first I would only mention technical stuff—which medicine I was currently taking, how it was administered, and its intended effect—before asking him about his day, what he was working on, what he'd had for lunch. But as the days of my cycle wore on, I became increasingly irritated. I'd had approximately three weeks of administering my own meds, of being solely responsible for reconstituting the powdered hormones at the prescribed amounts. Most difficult, both physically and psychically, was puncturing my own belly and ass with wide-gauge needles. (Needles, both in concept and in skin-puncturing action, made Gary queasy.) At about the same time, my mental focus shifted from the prosaic to the existential. I no longer cared about petty routines or politesse, what clothes I might put on in the morning, or whether a corporate client had praised Gary's lawyering skills. And hold out for an end-of-the-day exchange of niceties? Thank you, no.

Feverishly, I'd write down the questions that had kept me awake or had occurred to me on my way downtown for the writing classes I'd started taking. Standing outside the art school building, a prim Margaret Thatcher among the cigarette-smoking Mohawked and pierced, tattooed and bare-bellied, I searched the perimeter of the group for a decent cell zone from which to call Gary. El trains roared by as I dialed. Valerie, his assistant, picked up, and I shouted to be heard, apologizing for the noise and swearing I'd try to time my call better the next time. "Don't worry," she said. "There's always another one right behind it. It's great when you're running late and a complete headache otherwise. I think he's in his office. Hold on."

While Valerie buzzed Gary, I tried to picture him in his office, the small, low-ceilinged white room across the hall from the smoking lounge. I'd seen it only once, when he first moved in and needed my help arranging the too-large desk, file cabinet, and guest chair. When he made partner, I went to the flower shop for a congratulatory plant. I looked over the choices and contemplated an umbrella tree with spearmint-green leaves that the flower lady promised could withstand just about any conditions, a guarantee that made me nervous as I imagined how Gary might abuse this heartiness, pouring the remnants of morning cups of coffee into the soil or jotting reminders on the large tongue-shaped leaves. I considered an ornamental pepper, its quotation-mark-shaped fruits jutting up in perky phallic clusters. I worried that Gary might not like such an attention-grubbing specimen, this peacock of a plant. Finally I settled on a rubber tree and asked the delivery guy to please give the recipient explicit care instructions. "Don't assume he knows one thing about plant care," I said. "Please tell him about the water and the sunlight."

I'd ask after the tree, how it was doing, was it still alive. Gary thought it was.

"Are there green leaves on it?" I asked.

"I think so," he said. "Yeah, there are some. Near the top."

"Do you ever water it?"

"No," he said. "But maybe the cleaning crew does. I know someone's been picking up the dead leaves, and it certainly isn't me."

"Hello?" Gary answered on his speakerphone.

"It's me," I said, trying to modulate my volume so that Gary could hear me and the surrounding artistes could not. "Quick question. Do you think children who result from IVF are coincidental? A happy circumstance of our particular clinic, doctor, embryologist, and ultrasonographer, vials of Lupron and shots of Gonal-F? Or do you think they are timeless souls waiting for their most perfect embodiment?"

Gary picked up his phone and whispered, "Timeless souls."

"Thanks," I said, and hung up, looking around to see if anyone had heard. I didn't imagine these mostly younger students would know what I was talking about. Not like with normal overheard cell phone conversations, the guy in front of you at a crosswalk, speaking loudly into an ear-clip job, complaining about his boss or saying something you know to be false (his location, the start time of Sunday's Bears game, what makes a mole sauce a mole sauce) but recognize would be rude to correct. No, I figured, IVF probably meant little to my fellow students, unless it was also an acronym for something arty and cool, a digital art installation co-op or a human hair embroidery technique.

Corollary questions occurred to me. I was already late for class, and the last of the art school students were pushing through the smudged revolving door. I called Gary back. "Yes?"

he said, elongating and dipping the word in the middle so I'd know I was interrupting his work and testing his patience.

"Just to clarify, you think all babies, IVF and naturally occurring, are these timeless beings, their physical shape the only genetically influenced part? And are these timeless souls random ones, or do they descend exclusively from our ancestors? If ancestral, how are they divvied up among the children? Look how hard it is negotiating between our moms over where we spend Thanksgiving. To think our dead ancestors might also be jockeying for position."

"Hon, I appreciate how hard you're thinking about what we're doing, I really do. But I have a moot court in twenty minutes. Can we talk later, like at home tonight?"

"Promise you'll give it serious thought?" I asked.

"Promise," Gary said.

I sent him e-mails, articles on the potential risks of ART, others about heretofore infertile people conceiving, babies being born to a dead egg donor's sister, the custody battles of lesbian couples. Mostly, I sent more questions.

> Subject: Angst.
> G,
> You say souls are timeless, but where's the proof? Why would you say they are timeless when you're even more of a realist than I, putting aside your belief that I'm going to hell because I occasionally enjoy pork and believe religious dietary restrictions to be an archaic holdover from less sanitary times. By the way, the blackened catfish you like so well is unkosher, and that one is for good reason. Bottom feeder, yech.
> Love,
> Me

Subject: Re: Angst

Beth,

You are going to hell. And it'll be especially hellish because not only will you have an eternity of the usual hell stuff—fiery pits and pitchforks, Hitler and Jeffrey Dahmer—but because there'll be no pigs in hell, vilified on earth as they've been by the Jews and Muslims. By the way, the last time I checked, catfish are still fish. Not pigs. Not horses or whatever other animals the rabbis specify, but fish, as in Gefilte.

Your Loving Husband

As the weeks passed, it became nearly impossible for us to talk about anything without me turning it into something deep, heavy, freaky. This gravitas reminded me of college, my earnest self nestled in a beanbag chair in somebody's dorm room, passing around a bong plastered with band stickers. On Friday nights I'd hang out in the room of this guy at the end of the hall, talking about the Sandinistas, migrant workers' shameful living conditions, and the tattered ozone layer. The room would be packed, filled with UW Badgers waiting for their turn with the The Smiths bong, so enormous only the T and s dipped out of one's bleary-eyed, head-on view. But as serious as the issues we discussed, as many Fridays as I'd spent in there, these conversations were easy. We were strident, solid in our convictions, and knew that however tragic, Nicaragua and fruit farms and the stratosphere were a bazillion miles away from the warmth of our dorm, the coziness of our student union.

My current crop of issues was dead serious and deadly intimate. Older now, and sobered, I was being forced to reconsider my assumptions—about my health and my religion, about God, romance, and the meaning of life. Perhaps polycystic ovaries were just the tip of some disordered iceberg, I worried, and I had a mother lode of abnormalities lying in hibernation:

a miscarriage problem that wouldn't be discovered until the IVF succeeded, rheumatoid arthritis just beginning to lick at my joints, a dowager's hump that would eventually punctuate my seventy-year-old back.

I considered Stephen Hawking. Confined to a wheelchair since his twenties, unable to talk without a speech synthesizer, still he had sorted through the laws governing the universe. He rose above his dramatically earthbound self to shine brilliant lights on the infinite and cosmic, on space-time and black holes. He had never been well coordinated, he admits, and was neither athlete nor calligrapher; his strength had always been intellectual. Tragic as his motor neuron disease is, he still leads a fulfilling life. In addition to his spectacular mind, reputation, and career, he has a wife, children, and grandchildren. He says he feels complete.

With my polycystic ovaries, I worried I was doomed to a depthless life, that I'd die with my mothering strength un-tapped and my life purpose unfulfilled. My raison d'être might very well be to bunt, to generate the child who would cure can-cer, quell trouble in the Middle East, help the Cubs win a World Series. If I failed to have the child I was fated to have, if I had done something to screw up divine intention (could hu-man behavior trump divine intention?) and IVF didn't work, then I'd be nothing, have nothing. I'd go through the trouble and expense of IVF and end up with nothing to show for it but heartbreak, a ravaged reproductive system, and scars in the crooks of my arms like track marks.

I wanted to see into the future, to skip ahead to the end of my fertility story to know how it would turn out. I also had a strong impulse to divine any latent physical impairments. ART was spoiling me, making me believe any scientific inquiry was possible. In this age of MRIs that can reveal thought patterns and DNA configurations that lay bare genetic inheritance, one's physical self was ultimately knowable, if one were com-fortable with the knowledge and the means for acquiring it.

ART offers the chance to perform preimplantation genetic diagnosis (PGD) on an embryo by removing one or two cells at the four-to-ten-cell stage of development and analyzing the genetic material. It is used for a few purposes: to check for altered genes that could lead to one of dozens of inherited diseases, to select embryos that will be a matched tissue donor for an ailing sibling, to detect specific physical characteristics, or to determine sex. PGD is a thrilling scientific accomplishment and, if used to prevent disease or physical impairment, a boon to humankind. But it gave me the creeps. I pictured American minivans teeming with Nazi archetypes, Indian kindergarten classes without a single girl. Still, to get me past my anxiety and the suspense, I wanted to pluck out some of my genetic material—a couple of eyelashes or bits of cuticle—hand it over to the experts, and receive a full report about my present condition and what was to come.

I looked into getting a full body scan, this high-tech hunt for lurking problems, unruptured aneurysms, say, cancerous cells, or arterial plaque. The arguments for doing it were hard to ignore. One article quoted a doctor who had scanned tens of thousands of patients and had not encountered that single human being without some evolving pathology. He spoke of giving these patients the tools to tackle a still-preventable problem and of helping them feel as if they had greater control over their own bodies.

But other articles, the EPA, the FDA, the American College of Radiology, and the American Medical Association, to name a few, warned that preventive CT scans were so risky as to outweigh the benefits. The incidence of false positives was high; serious health problems were missed; and inconclusive results were common. Moreover the psychological burden for a person with potential abnormalities can be overwhelming. The amount of radiation is also not insignificant. As one radiologist put it, "An individual undergoing this examination receives much more radiation than they would from all other sources

for several years—they might as well take a trip to Chernobyl."
So why create another thing to be anxious about? Why undergo one more possibly risky medical procedure?

Gary and I stopped trying to discuss issues of substance—they
made me too crazy, and wordless activities, such as exercise
or sex, were difficult since I was often tender, my heretofore tucked-back and taken-for-granted innards a minefield of
swollen and painful obstacles. Thus began the period of our
marriage that I remember as the Acquaintanceship. Even
more than when we first began dating, our conversations now
centered on the topical and superficial, on severe weather
events and celebrity gossip. We tried spending our evenings
watching TV, but I could no longer abide the prevailing flip-
pancy on the sitcoms, and I wept inappropriately, copiously,
and at random during the dramas. Gary worried about me,
about us. He wanted to be of help, but I was becoming too
much for him to handle. I was becoming too much for Freud
or FEMA to handle. I made a conscious decision to look to experts for answers—to clergy, bioethicists, my mother.
    I called the Archdiocese of Chicago. Turns out they have a
whole department, the Respect Life Office, devoted to transforming "society into a Culture of Life where every human being is valued and protected from the moment of conception
until natural death." A woman answered, and I said hello, uncertain how to warm up to my subject, uncertain even what
my specific question was. We chatted a bit, about how once,
when the streets were really icy, I had slid right into Cardinal
Francis George as he was exiting the archdiocese building.
"He's a very patient man," the Respect Life woman said. "I'm
sure he wasn't bothered. So what can I do for you?"
    I explained that I was doing a bit of research about infertility
treatments. Truth was, I was going through in vitro fertilization

myself and had some questions that I thought might be outside my doctor's purview.

"Well. First off, while the Catholic Church does condone many fertility procedures, IVF is not one of them. It is immoral because it degrades the human being at so many levels—the husband and wife going through it, the extra embryos that are discarded or experimented on, et cetera. And often donor eggs or sperm are used, meaning a genetic parent is from outside the marriage, in clear violation of God's law. Also, because in vitro fertilization frequently causes a woman to become pregnant with more babies than she wished for, doctors reduce that number through abortion. You know how these so-called fetal reductions are brought about, don't you?"

"No, not really," I said.

"A syringe is filled with potassium chloride, and using ultrasound, the baby or babies that have somehow been determined to be less desirable have that needle plunged into their hearts. Sometimes the babies that are chosen are not necessarily less healthy, which is often trotted out as the rationale for these procedures. Sometimes they're selected simply because they're the easiest for the doctor to reach."

"God," I said, and immediately regretted saying, knowing the Respect Life office is also a Respect God office. "That is just awful. Of course I would never kill a perfectly fine baby. But I don't understand why, if my husband and I don't use any donor material, IVF would be considered immoral."

"In the first place, at the risk of being graphic, the way clinics ask the husbands to produce their sperm sample is already a prohibited offense against God. But there is an even greater sin here. IVF perverts the marital act from one of love into a manufacturing process, the children reduced to mere product. This brings me to my point. Like Jesus, human beings are begotten, not made—an incredibly important concept. Begotten, not made."

"Hmm. All right. Thank you so much," I said.

"By the way," she said, "this might make you feel better. Most Catholics aren't aware of the Church's stance on IVF. They don't realize that it, among other infertility treatments, is immoral. The good news for you is, if a couple is unaware that IVF is sinful, they are not subjectively guilty of sin. You are Catholic, right?"

"Yes," I said, bearing false witness. "Thanks again."

I looked up "begotten not made." It comes from the Nicene Creed used at Holy Mass, which states, "We believe in one Lord, Jesus Christ, the Only Son of God eternally begotten of the Father . . . begotten, not made, one in Being with the Father." According to Catholic.net, "the term 'begotten not made' means that the Second Person does not proceed from the First Person by creation. When a human being is conceived, the body comes from the father and the mother; the soul is created immediately from nothing by God."

Dozens of theology websites, I discovered, discuss issues surrounding ART and bioethics. Many started off by making clear the biblical importance of differentiated sexes and the clear connection between the two distinct sexes and procreation. They mentioned the strain that reproductive technology had placed on the connection between the sexual relationship of a man and woman and the birth of a child, how it had introduced production as the primary goal of procreation and deemphasized the mystery of the child who incarnates his parents' union.

In a paper called "Begotten Not Made: A Catholic View of Reproductive Technology," Dr. John Haas, president of the National Catholic Bioethics Center in Boston, reiterated the things I had heard from the Respect Life lady, about human beings making love, not babies, and how the marital act was no manufacturing process, the resulting children no products. "Like the Son of God himself," Haas writes, "we are the kind of beings who are 'begotten, not made' and, therefore, of equal status and dignity with our parents." Dr. Haas finds it troubling that in their very creation, IVF children are subjected to the arbitrary choices of the people working on their development. In violation of Church doctrine, they are treated not as human beings but as goods.

In 1987, the Sacred Congregation for the Doctrine of the Faith, the body charged by the Catholic Church "to promote and safeguard the doctrine on the faith and morals throughout the Catholic world," issued a document known as *Donum Vitae* (The Gift of Life), which addressed the morality of modern fertility treatments. The document did not say that using technology to overcome infertility was wrong in and of itself. Rather, it judged some methods to be moral and others, like those that harm the dignity of the human person or the institution of marriage, immoral. *Donum Vitae* teaches that "if a given medical intervention helps or assists the marriage act to achieve pregnancy, it may be considered moral: if the intervention replaces the marriage act in order to engender life, it is not moral."

In vitro fertilization is one such immoral procedure, says *Donum Vitae*, "because it eliminates the marriage act as the means of achieving pregnancy, instead of helping it achieve this natural end." IVF is a problem for a few reasons. First, it engenders new life not through an act of love between married people but by a lab procedure, reducing husband and wife to mere providers of necessary raw material. Second, it brings several embryos into existence, which is a terrible offense against human life, and the successful birth of one life at the expense of so many others is a great sin. *Donum Vitae* asserts, "The connection between in vitro fertilization and the voluntary destruction of human embryos occurs too often. This is significant: through these procedures, with apparently contrary purposes, life and death are subjected to the decision of man, who thus sets himself up as the giver of life and death by decree."

But the Catholic Church approves of "moral" interventions to overcome infertility, such as surgery to overcome tubal blockages and lower tubal ovum transfer, in which a wife's egg is repositioned beyond a tubal blockage to make it more accessible to the husband's sperm. But other techniques, such as gamete intrafallopian transfer (GIFT), dwell in a moral no-man's-land. GIFT involves removing the eggs from a ripened follicle and, via laparoscopy, placing them and some sperm in the fallopian tube. For the Catholic Church to approve of GIFT, the genetic material must belong to the husband and wife undergoing the intervention, and the sperm must be collected following "the marital act." Some theologians reject the procedure altogether as an immoral substitute for the marital act. Others see it as assisting the marital act and therefore permissible. The pope and bishops have not made any final judgment, so Catholic couples are still free to choose or reject GIFT depending on their own consciences. When and if the Church deems it to be immoral, however, GIFT should no longer be used. The children who have already resulted from successful rounds of GIFT will be grandfathered into heaven, one presumes.

Like so many troubled souls before me, I looked to the Bible for some clarity, flipping through to find the stories of fertility struggles and marital sex. Surprisingly, the Bible portrays sex as integral to the human experience, an essential part of the total context of human nature and happiness, a key component of marital companionship and not just a means to a procreative end. And according to Jewish law, a married couple can have sex in any way they wish so as to maximize their physical pleasure.

I checked out *Song of Solomon*, a cycle of poems about erotic love in the form of a dialogue between a bride and bridegroom. Peppered with explicit language and imagery, at least in a pre–*Girls Gone Wild* sense, it begins, "Let him kiss me with the kisses of his mouth!" a line that moved me, reminding me that people have been kissing since time immemorial, and that I hadn't been kissed—I mean really kissed, in more than just a chaste next-to-the-mouth-hello-or-goodbye-have-a-good-day-at-work way—for over a month.

The poems alternate between the groom and the bride's perspective. He says, "Your channel is an orchard of pomegranates with all choicest fruits." She says, "I had put off my garment; how could I put it on again? I had bathed my feet; how could I soil them? My beloved thrust his hand into the opening, and my inmost being yearned for him. I arose to open to my beloved, and my hands dripped with myrrh, my fingers with liquid myrrh." He says, "You are stately as a palm tree, and your breasts are like its clusters. I say I will climb the palm tree, and lay hold of its branches." I could tell these were newlyweds, young lovers. Give them a couple of years together, and I'll bet the bridegroom is comparing his wife's body parts to raisins, figs, and prunes.

I was in good company, as far as frustrated infertile wives go. In the Old Testament story of Elkanah and Hannah, Elkanah asks, "Hannah, why do you weep? And why do you not eat? And why is your heart so sad? Am I not more to you than ten sons?" Hannah clearly did love her husband but grieved at her inability to bear their children. I could relate. I did love my husband, thought he was the greatest in many regards—his sense of humor and work ethic, his ambition and appetite, the way he climbed my palm tree—but since having a baby was now my primary focus, and since the strength of his seed wasn't going to do the trick, his love suddenly seemed beside the point.

The Bible describes Sarah right off the bat as barren, a particularly significant descriptor since God had promised her husband, Abraham, that his children would become a great nation. For ten years she did not conceive (making our modern standard, that one year of unprotected sex without conception constitutes a fertility problem, seem downright hasty). Sarah then loaned Abraham her maid, Hagar, as a concubine (making our modern standard of medicalized treatments seem downright tolerable, from a female perspective). Hagar conceived and gave birth to Ishmael, a son for eighty-six-year-old Abraham. Thirteen years later, when Abraham was ninety-nine, God promised that he and Sarah, then ninety, would have a child, despite their advanced ages. A year later Isaac was born.

In the New Testament, John the Baptist's parents, Zechariah and Elizabeth, were "upright in the sight of God. But they had no children because Elizabeth was barren." These biblical tales with their happy endings, no matter how tortuous the wait, demonstrate that the final ability to have children is a sign of God's grace, that he bestows special favor on his elect. Modern medicine was nowhere in sight, and still these fantastic results! These *alter kockers* with their apparently uneventful pregnancies and childbirths, their ability to get it on at advanced ages—the risk of broken hips or pneumonia taken in youthful stride—the lack of Viagra and K-Y, these prosthetic methods for extending one's potent youth a nonissue, back in the days of yore. Talk about your biblical miracles!

Where had these prosaic wonders gone? More important, where had the Bible's interactive God gone? Back then He was constantly involved, sending messages to this one to sacrifice his son and that one to take dictation. Putting aside the Virgin Mary–pictorial grilled cheese sandwiches and Jesus on a Chihuahua's ear, the pope's-mitre Dorito chips and Our Lady of Guadalupe sap on a tree stump, where was God on earth? And what was the best way to reach Him? Could He read my thoughts? Would telepathic messages sent from my family room suffice? Or did I have to speak out loud, go to an official holy place, eat certain foods, wear certain vestments, make a pilgrimage, and utter specific prayers in a specific order?

Occasionally I'd encounter appeals to God and religious invocations around the fertility clinic, cross charms dangling from necklaces, Jewish stars and other holy accessories glinting in the fluorescent light. Infertility isn't an incurable disease per se, but according to a 2003 *Newsweek* poll, 72 percent of Americans say they believe praying to God can cure a person, even a medically terminal one. On the popular interfaith website called Beliefnet, the vast majority of the 35,000 prayer circles are health related. The way it works is, anyone, whether acquainted with the patient or merely a compassionate stranger, can log on and offer their virtual prayers to heal, cure, and combat illness and disability, taking the mixing of technology and religion just one step further.

It unsettled me, this indiscriminate flitting between modern medicine and religion. I don't mean my fellow patients' faith in both science and God—I understand how faith and spirituality can counteract stress and despair, perhaps contributing to a better scientific outcome. But they seemed to believe that medicine was good only up to a certain point and that, from that point on, they'd surrender themselves to God, a faith that struck me as arbitrary, reductive, and vain. Was there some precise moment at which God would take over, breathing His magic into the burgeoning His Likenesses? How were these people to know when they'd reached that stage? Perhaps the doctor attempting to examine the patient now under God's care would receive a shock. Or maybe God would give a shout out to the doctors, using the technology as His conduit, posting messages or sacred images on the sonogram, a glowing Jesus on the Cross filling the uterine cavity, praying hands in the general area of the bladder.

Perhaps it was more of an atelier-model, with God as the maestro under whose direction a bunch of sous-chefs, in the form of medical personnel, scurried to carry out the messy and tedious prep work. But I struggled with the idea that God just stood by, waiting to be needed like so much tech support. Even if He was responsible for creating human beings who had the capability and wherewithal to develop the procedures and medication to accomplish reproductive feats, certainly He didn't wait around for each individual patient to summon Him when she hit a physical or moral dead end.

A 2005 *New York Times* article addressed this tension between God and science by looking into the religiosity of scientists. Some scientists argue that belief in God and faith in science are irreconcilable, that religion is nothing more than "magical thinking." Others believe science and religion are two separate realms, "nonoverlapping magisteria," as Stephen Jay Gould, the late evolutionary biologist, called them. According to Gould, science holds sway in the realm of "what the universe is made of (fact) and why does it work this way (theory)," while religion trumps science on "questions of meaning and moral value." But others voice their dissatisfaction with this model, believing that scientists' moral values inevitably influence their work and that much of science carries ethical implications out into the real world.

More and more scientists, according to the article, are now reconciling their dual faiths. Not only are they challenging the religious view that scientists are secular elitists and science is godless, but they feel, through observation and study, that nature and science go only so far to explain human beings—their behavior and their physical makeup. Dr. Francis S. Collins, a scientist and a Christian, says, "You will never understand what it means to be a human being through naturalistic observation. You won't understand why you are here and what the meaning is. Science has no power to address those questions—and are they not the most important questions we ask ourselves?" Dr. Collins makes a compelling argument, but examined ideas are quite a different thing from the confusion I saw around me.

The Iowa couple who gave birth to septuplets in 1997, Bobbi and Kenneth McCaughey, emphasized that God was responsible for their seven babies. But science and technology had enabled their conception, yielding a pregnancy that resembled not a biblical one but a dog's or a cat's. Born nine weeks early, the babies spent months in the hospital. When they finally came home, Bobbi McCaughey said, "Nothing's going to happen today that God hasn't already planned for me." Kenneth McCaughey added, "God has told us that He won't give us more than we can handle. And on the other side of that, God wants to handle our problems for us."

But hadn't their infertility also been God's will? How were the McCaugheys certain that the doctors weren't somehow messing up God's plan, trampling all over His turf with their man-made medicine and institutional procedures? As Diana Butler Bass, a religion professor, wrote in *The New York Times*, "If the McCaugheys thought about it, they might notice a glaring inconsistency in their actions. If the existence of seven embryos is God's will, then why didn't Bobbi McCaughey accept her own infertility as God's will? Since she and her husband could not have children without the aid of drugs, perhaps it was God's will to remain childless. But no. The McCaugheys could not believe that, so they sought science to help God accomplish a divine plan."

Perhaps my access to modern science had jaded me, left me viewing the world through petri-dish lenses, but without the science, I found it impossible to believe that any of these people stood a chance. The Hannahs and Sarahs and Elizabeths with their aged eggs and their husbands' senior sperm; the Bobbi McCaugheys with the seven newborns who had required a team of sixty doctors to help them at birth, nature just does not work this way. Yes, miraculous fertility stories do occur—the woman who undergoes multiple rounds of IVF for a first, hard-won pregnancy, then becomes unexpectedly and quickly pregnant on her own the second time; the fifty-year-old woman who conceives without medication; the families with a couple of sets of naturally occurring twins; the couples who give up trying to get pregnant and adopt a baby, only to realize they're pregnant. But I'm chalking these up as anomalies, not actual superhuman occurrences.

As for ninety- and hundred-year-old women conceiving— well, what with all the difficulties that women past the age of thirty-five have, it's enough to make the faithful ask some questions. By the time a woman reaches her twenties, her fertility is already beginning its descent, and a particularly sharp drop occurs in the mid- to late thirties. Experts believe that by the age of forty-three, a woman has less than a 5 percent chance of getting pregnant on her own. True, our modern world differs from the biblical one, with its industrial, scientific, and technological advances, the varieties of beer, and the sheer fact of pants. But the body's basic functions remain the same. And even if fifty is the new thirty, that would make ninety only the new seventy—way too late to be having a child, from a physical (and sociological and tranquil-twilight-years) standpoint.

Even without the medical complication of advanced age, it seems to this technology-keen mother that gestating women in the Bible were largely in the medical dark. If complications came up in conceiving, carrying the baby to term, or delivering it safely, a woman had little recourse but to seek the help of experienced people, secure for herself a particularly well-whittled birthing stool, or pray, pray, pray. Sure, the midwife scene was better back then. But if I'm choosing between an experienced birth attendant and a university-trained surgeon to get the breech baby with his umbilical cord wrapped around his neck safely out of me and into the world, I'm choosing the surgeon every time.

Maybe biblical years differed from the modern 365-day standard; a simple math problem with years accounting for fewer days, back in the day. Maybe biblically hundred-year-old new moms were really in their mid-thirties—older, yes, but certainly not ancient. Or maybe the numbers are not meant to be taken literally. Maybe their meaning derives from their context; if Moses was said to die at the age of 120, then all significant events were to be viewed through the filter of a 120-year lifespan. Perhaps the Bible is a collection of parables, creation stories with symbolic importance but intentionally simplified to make clear their morals. I understood the point of the fertility stories: I was supposed to put aside my ego, my ultimately powerless human efforts, and trust in God; I was to understand that perhaps I'd transgressed and that the answer to my barrenness would be to pray. But I was still troubled, uncertain how to face whatever issues were still to come and skeptical about the power of prayer to help. How should a truly faithful infertility patient, one who revels in the medicine and also asks God for strength, who follows the doctor's instructions and also fasts on Yom Kippur, negotiate between the human and the divine?

My rabbi back then was a conservative Jew with strong opinions on most issues. When I checked in with him he was only too happy to talk, explaining that more and more he was being forced to question himself and his accepted beliefs and to look to the Talmud and rabbinic texts about where Judaism draws the line on assisted reproduction. He had noticed a dramatic uptick in the number of his congregants facing infertility and grappling with the issues it raises, and he wondered whether the Jewish community had a higher incidence of fertility problems than the population at large. He was onto something. Jews and Asians, studies suggest, are more likely to have trouble getting pregnant. Michael Gold, author of *And Hannah Wept*, confirms this observation: while 15 to 20 percent of all American couples of childbearing age are clinically infertile, he says, the percentage of infertile Jewish couples is higher. "The reason is simple," he writes. "Jews tend to marry later and postpone having children longer than the general population. They tend to go to college, to be attracted to the professions, and to spend several years in the graduate programs that lead into those professions. More Jewish women are remaining in the workforce and delaying the decision to have children as long as possible. When educational and professional commitments come first, women usually wait until their thirties to begin childbearing."

All three branches of Judaism permit artificial insemination, but only after the couple explores the alternatives. Donor material, however, is a source of disagreement, particularly when the donor is a non-Jew. To the extent that masturbation is prohibited, an exception is generally made for the purpose of sample collection. Fetal reduction, like abortion generally, is permitted under certain circumstances, such as when a pregnancy poses a realistic threat to the mother's life or the fetus is nonviable. Judaism refers to the threatening fetus as a *rodef*, or pursuer, of the mother's life. But when a reduction is to be performed for the sake of the remaining fetuses' health, when the fetuses are *rodfim* or pursuers of one another, Jewish law is less clear. Some rabbis say it depends on the age of the fetuses, since the Talmud refers to fetuses before the fortieth day of gestation as "mere water." Others say it is against Talmudic law to choose one life over any others. In any case, fetal reduction is never allowed for personal convenience or as a matter of choice, such as to reduce twins to a singleton. The permissibility of purposefully implanting multiple embryos in the first place is itself seriously questionable, since the difficult situation of multiple gestations could likely result.

I asked Rabbi Schachter whether he considered IVF moral. The first commandment in the Torah, he said, is to be fruitful and multiply, and when couples had difficulty conceiving on their own, assisted reproduction was therefore permitted. Not only did assisted reproductive technologies uphold the Talmudic imperative to sanctify life, they built upon it and illustrated to people the miracle and immeasurable value of human life.

Maimonides, the twelfth-century Jewish philosopher and medical text writer, said that "whoever adds even one Jewish soul is considered as having created an entire world."

"That's a lot of pressure," I said. "Is there a negative equivalent? I mean, is it some sort of sin for Jews not to have kids?"

Rabbi Schachter explained that by Jewish law, a married man must have at least two children. "The Mishnah claims that the married man is subject to the biblical commandment to procreate and that to fulfill this holy duty, he must father at least two children. So in our day and age, when increasing numbers of people are having difficulty conceiving, it is clear that technologies that assist in conception are considered moral, within boundaries."

I worried I'd be the reason my straight-as-an-arrow, do-gooder husband would get in spiritual trouble. The Tosefta (a second compilation of oral law, which serves as a supplement to the Mishnah, the first recording of oral law of the Jewish people) rules that a man who has no children may not serve as a judge; presumably his lack of experience with children renders him insufficiently appreciative of their importance. Any accused person is somebody's child, the reasoning goes, and if the death penalty is in the offing, the judge must be sensitive to what is at stake.

This information weighed me down. Archaic or not, I related to the rationale: judges should be well-rounded, empathic people, able to understand and deconstruct individual cases in a thoughtful, informed way. I also understood the importance of repopulating the world, even in the face of global overpopulation. But I didn't want to place Gary's spiritual afterlife in jeopardy. More important, I didn't want Gary's judicious temperament and impeccable legal training to be wasted simply because I couldn't have his babies. He'd gone to Stanford Law, graduating at the tippy-top of his class, and then clerked for an extraordinary federal court of appeals judge and afterward for a Supreme Court justice. He'd made partner at a blue-chip law firm and was building a reputation as a brilliant yet likable litigator. He was perfect judge material, except for this one flaw—a polycystic, anovulatory wife threatening to fuck up his excellent résumé. And even if he didn't care what Jewish law had to say about how he navigated the American legal system, I regretted the shadow of doubt I was casting.

IVF, Rabbi Schachter explained, resembled other scientific feats that improved the human condition by healing, ameliorating suffering, or helping to fulfill commandments. It was therefore not just okay but a blessing. He warned, however, that specific procedures or iterations were on shaky moral ground, and that when third parties were involved, genetically or otherwise, one had to be extra vigilant to keep the Laws of Torah in mind. Reform Jews generally allow surrogate pregnancy but emphasize the importance of using the couple's own eggs and sperm. Then Rabbi Schachter told me about a couple, congregants, both Jewish, who had gone through IVF and implanted their fertilized embryos in a Gentile gestational surrogate. When the baby was born, Rabbi Schachter had insisted upon a *mikvah* (a purifying bath).

"But the baby was Jewish," I said. "Genetically Jewish with traceable roots. His parents were standing right there when he was born. Genetic testing would have linked them directly up."

"It doesn't matter. The Talmud recognizes motherhood through parturition, or birth. The woman carrying and birthing the child is therefore considered its mother. And Judaism is matrilineal, the religion of the mother determining the child's. Therefore, non-Jewish surrogate, technically non-Jewish baby. That's why we went to the *mikvah*. We purified the baby, symbolically washing away the nine months in the surrogate's body, symbolically making him his parents. I also didn't want there to be any question about whether the child was Jewish when it came time to, say, think about marriage to a more conservative Jew."

"But he was his parents', genetically and in every other way."

"We're talking about Jewish law, right? Not about what your first instincts might be. There is a difference. And anyway, many interpreters of Jewish law would still have considered the child non-Jewish, since his gestation runs counter to Talmudic law. The Talmud makes clear that surrogacy is not permitted. In the first place, it is a form of prostitution: money tendered, body sacrificed. Second, it creates a situation in which a woman exposes herself to physical and emotional harm, and that is explicitly forbidden. Finally, a gestational relationship is also a biological relationship is also a legal relationship, according to Jewish law. It's quite complicated and oftentimes at odds with American law."

We discussed Jewish law as it relates to maternity and paternity, particularly in cases involving artificial insemination or sperm donorship. Would using donor sperm, even sperm acquired through a Jewish sperm bank, be considered wrong somehow, either adulterous or unkosher? Rabbi Schachter got up, went to his bookshelf, and fetched *Matters of Life and Death: A Jewish Approach to Modern Medical Ethics* by Elliot Dorff, chair of bioethics at the University of Judaism in Los Angeles. Dorff writes, "Physicians report that while traditional Jews who use DI (donor insemination) prefer non-Jewish donors for fear of incest in the next generation, liberal Jews want Jewish donors. The motivations for that tendency may be many, but undoubtedly for some people insemination by a non-Jew smacks of intermarriage, and others probably hold an ethnic notion of Jewish identity." Dorff goes on to discuss the rationale of using non-Jewish donors to safeguard health, such as guarding against Jewish genetic diseases.

Rabbi Michael J. Broyde, who teaches Jewish law at Emory University School of Law, wrote an article entitled "The Establishment of Maternity and Paternity in Jewish and American Law." Many rabbis, he states, consider genetic relationship to be the sole determinant of paternity. Therefore a sperm donor (a medical procedure that is more than fifteen hundred years

old, judging from the fact the Babylonian Talmud mentions artificial insemination as a possibility) has paternity rights.

But rabbis disagree over what this means. Some believe that
insemination using donor sperm is allowed, while others consider it an act of adultery. Rabbi Broyde says that some rabbis
believe that genetically mixing a donor's sperm with a married
patient's egg is not an act of adultery, but that injecting such
sperm during an insemination procedure is physically analo-
gous to an adulterous act, and is therefore a prohibited form of
adultery. Others also believe the procedure violates the rules of
modesty. Finally, Rabbi Y. Breish thinks that heterologous insemination (or donor insemination, as opposed to homologous
insemination, or insemination using the husband's sperm) is
not an adulterous act but that "from the point of view of our religion these ugly and disgusting things should not be done, for
they are similar to the deeds of the land of Canaan and its
abominations."

As for maternity, Jewish law states that it is a matter of genetics and biology. If conception occurs in one woman, and then
the fetus is implanted in another, the place of conception es-
tablishes the first woman's motherhood. But if an in vitro conception occurs, Jewish law focuses on birth as establishing
motherhood.

Another rabbi I know chuckled when I asked him about the
current Jewish stance not only on the historical accuracy of the
Bible, but also on IVF and other assisted reproductive technologies. "There's an old saying," he said. "Maybe you've
heard it. It goes, show me three Jews and I'll show you five
opinions."

He cautioned me to keep in mind that the Bible represents
a patriarchal model, that back in that time, if a couple failed to
conceive within seven years, it was assumed to be the wife's
fault and the man could take another wife. After polygamy was
outlawed in the Middle Ages, and actually until fairly recently,

he would be allowed to divorce her in order to remarry a pre-sumably fertile new wife.

Meanwhile, I was holding out hope that one of my mom's fa-vorite palliative aphorisms would prove true. She had many of them: not only the one about the first child serving as guinea pig, but also ones about having tears at night but knowing there will be joy in the morning, and the healing benefits not only of food but of the soup variety, most especially her matzoh-balled version. In college I'd have occasional panic attacks and would call my mom to say how senseless it seemed. I labored all those years to learn to play the piano, speak French, and remember gymnastics routines, and now my current occupation— memorizing Turkish intellectual history—seemed moronic when we'd all be dead in a relatively short time anyway.

"A college education is not a waste of time," she'd say. "Knowledge about different cultures is not a waste of time. When you finish school, not only will you have a sense of self-satisfaction for all you learned, but you'll be more desirable on the job market and the person to sit next to at dinner parties. And what's with the negative attitude? Are you eating well? Getting enough sleep?"

"I'm fine, Mom. I just don't believe I'm going to get a great advertising job because of my knowledge of African folk tales. God, all the stuff I've crammed into my brain—Chaucer's *Canterbury Tales* in Old English, sonata after étude after rhap-sody, and now the life and times of Mustafa Kemal Atatürk. Not only will it not help me evade death, it will cease to exist when I do. A life's worth of esoterica filling a brain that will end up mushy at some point, a sieve for the information I've wasted my life trying to pack in. It's a cruel joke really and a huge waste of higher education dollars."

"Once you're a mother, you'll understand," she said. "I used to have those thoughts, too. But then you and Danny and David were born, and suddenly my life made sense. My days were fulfilled, and my life was validated. Once you kids took your first steps, I no longer worried about losing my own ability to walk. And as you've achieved various proficiencies and milestones, I've felt even more certain that my time on earth has been well spent. Honey, I have news for you. If you go through life being this vain, and I don't know what else to call your placing such a premium on yourself, you'll end up lonely and psychotic. I think you are wonderful and special, and you've helped make my life complete, but every person has their time, and once it's over, that's okay. In the meantime I feel good knowing that when I go, I'll be leaving a big part of myself behind—in my children and grandchildren's hearts and minds and in your physical selves. I'm also giving you my jewelry."

I continued having anxiety attacks, but rather than seeking help from one of the counselors at the student health center, I determined to try to control my own consciousness. After all, I figured, my thoughts about death weren't a sign of a mental problem or deep-rooted psychosis. To the contrary, they proved I was reflective and mentally robust, willing to seek out the darkest corners of my consciousness and unwilling to be distracted from profundity by material things, flashy entertainments, or partying.

And who knew—maybe my mother's not completely unbelievable explanation about children imbuing meaning would be the thing to do the trick. But what if I had kids who disappointed me, from a mental-health, essential-satisfaction standpoint? What if I had this perfect baby, nursed and potty-trained him, attended his football games and spelling bees, met his wife-to-be and danced at their wedding, and got to sit in while she gave birth and all that while, I'd be mentally counting down the years until my death. *If I'm thirty-three when I have a kid*, I'd think, *and people only live to be like eighty, even with medical advances, assuming I don't die early of a tragic accident or cancer (or malaria or the avian flu or a biological attack), I only have a handful of decades left. Only enough years to count on one hand, if I count in multiples of ten, which will fly since by thirty-three you've already been out of high school for fifteen years and it feels like only yesterday.*

I imagined my death and funeral, who would come, who would speak. I'd make sure to specify what outfit I wished to be buried in, and I wouldn't want an organ, preferring an acoustic guitar or straight-up piano. The mortician would prepare my body for interment, suctioning out all the tissue and blood and fat and pumping in the preservatives. Preservatives! After a lifetime spent trying to avoid those unhealthy fuckers! The body guy would be nonchalant, treating me like any other old female body to be dealt with, positioning the limbs I'd once been in control of, arranging the hair I should have been in control of. He'd finish the embalmment, dress me, and apply the wrong shade of lipstick. A job well done, with time to spare since he was extremely efficient, he'd pick up the clipboard attached to the foot of the stainless-steel body-prep table and read a little about me. All my joints and teeth were original, but my uterus and ovaries had been removed following ovarian cancer linked to massive doses of hormones during my child-bearing years, which had stretched on for nearly a decade, yielding the seven children I'd kept having in hopes that the next one would trigger my mother's promised soporific.

7

Nonindigenous Plants

Once you've traveled fifteen miles north of Chicago, the single-family homes lining the highway's eastern edge give way to forested stretches reminiscent of northern Wisconsin. I fantasize that Gary and I are driving to a rented cabin Door County–way for a weekend of ice fishing, cross-country skiing, sharp cheddar fondue, and fireplace-warmed lovemaking. I've been tracking my menstrual cycle and in exactly five and a half hours I'll release an egg from my lucky right ovary. After a day spent gamboling in the brisk northern air, we'll come inside, light a fire, sip cognac, and watch the sun set. I'll take a hot shower and close my eyes, waiting for the barely perceptible pinch, a buried reminder of my womanliness and the miracle of human procreation, this automatic and reliable inheritance. I'll pat dry my well-functioning body, anoint it with musky oils, and summon Gary to the furry rug spread before the hearth.

Weekend well spent, we'll drive home, and for the next ten days I'll go about my business knowing intuitively that I am with child. Examining packages of boneless, skinless chicken breasts, ordering books of stamps, I'll be focused inward, even as my glow emanates out to the world. On the eleventh day I'll administer a home pregnancy test. The result window will immediately turn hot, hot pink, setting all sorts of records for quickest and most undeniably positive result, which of course I won't realize, knowing only that it works just like they say it will on TV.

I'll bake chocolate soufflés and nestle the test stick inside Gary's serving, spooning extra whipped cream on top. First we'll sup on trout and fiddlehead ferns, and then I'll serve dessert. Gary'll sink a spoon into the ramekin, feel it thump against something unexpectedly nonfudgy, scoop out the test, and lick the plastic stick clean. He will neither question what he is looking at nor, upon realizing how those things work, say a word about having ingested my urine. He'll simply revel in the knowledge that his beautiful, sexy, womanly, perfectly fecund wife is having his baby. His eyes will glisten, and wordlessly, he'll guide me to our bed for some profoundly meaningful lovemaking.

"Mind if I turn this up?" Gary asks now, twisting the radio volume dial. *But I'm too full to swallow my pride.* "Hey, there's a cop over there on the shoulder, and this song is by the Police. Good omen." *I can't stand losing you. I can't stand losing youououou.*

"What are you talking about? It's not an omen. It's called a coincidence and not a very significant one. Who cares about the Police? What do police of any sort have to do with my getting pregnant? If it were, I don't know, Genesis—that *would* be kind of cool. Urge Overkill. The Sex Pistols. Barenaked Ladies. Chubby Checker even. But the Police? How about Bachman-Turner Overdrive, Gar? Would that trip you out, man? Would it prove God's existence or send you a clear signal that today is the ideal time for some uterine strip-mining and clinical whacking off?"

"You're impossible."

"I know. Isn't that our real problem?"

"I have no idea how to answer that."

"Good," I say, "then don't. I just think that sometimes our bodies work in mysterious ways, and maybe your DNA objects to joining up with mine, and that's the source of our infertility. It knows a raving bitch who was never meant to have kids when it meets one."

"You're not a raving bitch, honey," Gary says, patting my sweat-panted knee. "Just raving."

Outside the window the implausibly robust trees, mostly evergreens, looking downright British Columbian in their perfect, conical, blue-green fir-ness, are somehow surviving, despite the sheer amount of exhaust they absorb day to day and the man-made tilt of the expressway bank. In fact, I am responsible for a good chunk of the exhaust they've absorbed lately. In the first two weeks of my cycle alone, I spent close to twenty IVF-related hours in my car. These weren't like the sexy, adrenaline-fueled road trips I took in college: heading southeast, Madison's domed capital building shrinking in my rearview mirror, while I traced circles on different boyfriends' hands as they shifted gears, racing at eighty-five miles per hour toward bands tuning up in dark Chicago clubs. These post-collegiate treks were torturous, slow-moving, isolated, pre-dawn, caffeine-*verboten* rigmaroles, WBBM informing me how fucked I was, weather- and traffic-wise, on the eights.

There were moments when I wanted to turn around, go back home, and try it again some other time, a response not to the IVF but to the bigger frustration, the omnipresent traffic. I'd call Gary, who'd remind me of Cara Alberts's advice, then chastise me for using my cell phone while driving and hang up.

"Ladies, avoid stress at all costs," Cara had said. "Stress destroys everything you're trying to achieve. I sometimes ask patients to think of stress as Pac-Man—remember that game from the video arcade?—and the eggs growing inside of you as those little dots Pac-Man feeds on. When you're feeling especially tired or irritable, or if you slice your finger opening a glass vial containing your medicine, or if you and your partner find yourself quarreling over piddly things, or if somebody cuts you off in traffic, remember this mantra that one of my patients used and that I find so lovely and instructive." She unfolded a piece of paper, put on her glasses, and read. "'I am at peace. I feel calm. I am trying to become a mother, to give birth to a new life precisely because all life is beautiful and all people miraculous. I choose to undergo infertility treatment because I love people and wish to create more of them. I will not let small obstacles derail me from my ultimate, wondrous goal.'"

Commune with your car, I think. *Commune with traffic. We're all in it together. I love you people and am desperate to make more just like you. You, sir. Yes, you, with the greasy mustache and "I ❤ Ass" bumper sticker. May God grant me sons just like you. You, too, ma'am, in the sparkly convertible. I admire the way you peer extra attentively at disabled vans and Cook County sheriffs writing up moving violations, the way you reduce your speed to ten miles per hour to ensure you won't miss observing slightly dented fenders or mild cases of whiplash. If I end up having a daughter, may she be every bit the bloodsucking tapeworm that you are.*

Four lanes of cars, trucks, and vans head north; the fifth, to the far left, is under construction, flushing the fast-lane regulars into the remaining road. They are the ones honking and giving the finger, yelling at Gary and calling him an asshole even though I, the most voluble of backseat drivers, can vouch for the fact that in this case he's done nothing wrong. We inch forward. Accelerator. Brake. Accelerator. Brake. We read people's vanity plates (X WIFE) and bumper stickers ("*If God*

Didn't Want Us to Eat Animals, He Wouldn't Have Made Them Out of Meat") and wish it were some other day, one with extra padding in the morning for sleeping in, sex, eggs, and newspapers.

"There's no such thing as a reverse commute," Gary observes. "Trite but true." The five lanes of traffic on the other side of the median, the tracks and the freezing CTA riders, snail their way south, toward the high-rises, the fluorescent-lit offices, and our rumpled, flannel-sheeted bed.

A Beanie Baby road show noses in front of us. I wonder if the stuffed-animal pyramid arranged on the car's back ledge belongs to kids, or if this is an adult collector. I determine never to buy juvenilia—stuffed animals or holiday-themed pencils or whimsical cupcakes—unless it is intended for real live children.

"Are you nervous?" Gary asks, braking.

"I don't know. Not really," I say. "I mean, no more than I've been the past month."

"But this is so much more important," Gary says. "And if it doesn't work out, I'd hate for you to have to go through it all again."

"If I have to, I will, and I don't want you telling me we shouldn't. I need your support."

"But it's a hassle for you and hard on both of us. And at ten thousand dollars a try, with like five thousand dollars' worth of medicine on top of that, it's a ton of money to throw at something that may never pan out."

"Gary. These are kids we're talking about. Not a craps game or a fantasy football league, but a statistically feasible medical procedure that might very well end in a pregnancy. Look, you're all I've got, and if you can't marshal some faith in IVF, try to rally around my enthusiasm for it. At the very least, couldn't you just pretend you think it'll work, you know, to prevent me from going into some sort of psychotic state? Couldn't you make like a humane and supportive partner and not give in to whatever compulsion you apparently feel to speak the terrifying and cruel truth? I have an idea—pretend I'm your chronically sick dog that you've decided to put down. Mislead me, but only because you love me and wish to protect me. So you'll tell me that we're just going for a ride, same as always, and then, when we get to the doctor and I begin to whimper, you'll remind me how many times I'd been there before and always well cared for. Then when they call my name, you'll give me a little pat and tell me it's okay. And when they lay me out on the cold examination table, you'll kiss the top of my head, and when the doctor says he's ready, you'll tell me it'll be okay, that pretty soon I'll be out of my misery and resting peacefully."

"You want me to lie to you?" Gary asks. "Is that what you're saying?"

"No. Not lie, exactly. Just throw me a line. You know, to prevent me from sinking completely. Or if that's too much to ask, at the very least maybe you could take your foot off the top of my head."

"I'm sorry. You've just been really confident, and I don't want to see you crushed if it doesn't happen."

"I have not been confident. Hopeful, yes. Excited about the prospect and amazed by the technology and happy with Hamlin, yes. But confident? I'd be the first to tell you there's no IVF guarantee. What are Hamlin's success rates, anyway? He claims they're slightly above average, so what, thirty-five percent per embryo transfer? That's hardly a sure thing. If somebody told you that your rubber had a thirty-five percent chance of preventing you from catching a hooker's syphilis, would you go ahead and take that chance? And since I've never been pregnant before—no abortions, no miscarriages to prove I can get there—who knows if I'm even capable? This is how I see it—we're these lunatic horticulturalists living in the Midwest but dead set on cultivating nonindigenous species in the inhospitable, arid soil of our sliver of urban backyard. We've done the footwork, tended the land, cut back any shady overhang, and fertilized the hell out of the dirt. We've found a reputable nursery that consistently grows hardy specimens, and we've done our best to transport and transplant the trees, not only in accordance with expert instructions but as to replicate their natural conditions."

"Weird. I just read an article on the invasion of nonindigenous plants as this grave threat to the integrity of the ecosystem. I think it was in *Harper's*."

"Are you doing this on purpose?"

"Doing what?" Gary sounds genuinely perplexed. "They're just really disruptive, that's all."

"Are you trying to make me feel like I'm wasting my time and endangering my body? Are you purposely acting like a moron to give me an alternate locus for my negative feelings? If so, on either point, mission accomplished. Excellent work."

"Again, I'm just trying to be the voice of reason. But I swear, I only mentioned it because it was a strange coincidence, your metaphor and this article I finished reading the other day. It might have been in the *Atlantic*, actually. I didn't mean to suggest anything by it—I'm just trying to have a conversation with my wife. But if I were to compare the IVF to something botanical—that's what you called us, crazy botanists, right?— I'd say it's more like planting a palm tree above the Arctic Circle and hoping for coconuts."

"You're right, Gary. That is better. Not only does it suggest that my uterus is inhospitable to life, it also manages to hint at my frigidity."

"Come on, honey. You are not frigid. In fact, you look great! Nice and curvy."

After telling Gary that my shape has nothing to do with whether I am or am not frigid, that the fact I didn't want him to touch me was the real indication, I ask him to please stop talking and chalk his negativity up to discomfort about having to produce a specimen. If only he'd prepared a little more for this day, I think, read the literature and looked through the guidelines, he'd know what to expect and not take out his distress on me. He'd be speechless as he agonized over what was to come.

I, on the other hand, had boned up on proper semen-collection techniques, both for my own edification and because I wanted to be able to offer Gary some professional pointers. Yet there never seemed a right time to bring it up. I hesitated, worried that I'd spook him or cause him to second-guess this thing I assumed he'd been ad-libbing for twenty-plus years. So I kept my mouth shut, even as I mentally scrolled through the instructions from both the informational packet and the sheet of paper stapled to the brown-paper lunch sack that Great Lakes Fertility sent home with me at my last appointment. They did this in case my partner couldn't accompany me the morning of my procedure, in which case he'd have to produce the specimen at home, placing me in charge not only of delivering my egg-full self but also of couriering Gary's spermy parcel to the clinic.

A sperm donor was to refrain from ejaculating from two to five days prior to producing the specimen, the instructions said, since longer or shorter periods of abstinence yield less healthy results. The time restriction had confused me. Which was it? Two days or five? How would a man know if he was a two- or five-dayer? Still, I regretted not having shared this crucial direction with Gary. I didn't know whether he'd done any ejaculating in the past few days, and I doubted I'd get an honest response if I asked. And anyway, it was too late now. Quite possibly the prime stuff had already been flushed, the grade-A sample now just like any other Lake Michigan flotsam, merging and hobnobbing with the gobs of E. coli and Enterococci.

I had also investigated the impact of mood and stress upon sperm quantity and quality. Evidence shows that stress negatively impacts quality, probably due to stress-induced hormonal changes. But even normal samples can contain some abnormal or dead sperm. In our case, Dr. Hamlin found that Gary's sample contained a slightly lower number of sperm than normal, and a slightly elevated number of abnormal sperm. But, he assured us, since a highly skilled technician would be sorting Gary's ejaculate, selecting one normal sperm and injecting it directly into the egg using ICSI, there'd be no problem—a few decent-looking buggers was all we'd need.

I worried that even with an expert's guiding hand, Gary's recent insensitivity might cause the gentle sperm to die off or transmute into abnormal types, their heads hanging and their tails between their phantom legs, leaving only a marauding pack of barracuda to attract the embryologist's eye. Once placed in the dish, they'd race straight toward the ova, swimming over one another and whipping one another with their slashing tails like little spermatozoan triathletes, burrowing in even before the embryologist could get them inside her needle, a raiding posse that would most certainly yield belligerent children.

Interestingly, evidence seems to debunk the notion that wearing boxer shorts or immersing the testicles in cold water improves semen quality, although either choice is okay, from a libertarian perspective. A research study from the Netherlands demonstrated that wearing tight leather trousers and tight plastic underpants together affected sperm motility, but neither had an effect on its own—good news for a husband of mine who shall remain nameless.

The specimen should be produced by masturbation, the instructions clarified, noting that neither oral stimulation nor coitus interruptus was acceptable. *Wash your genitals and hands. Many materials are toxic to sperm, and most contain contaminants, so use only the sterile container provided. Swab penis tip with enclosed medi-wipe, washing outward from the meatus toward the sulcus. Place sterile container close to glans to assure complete catch. Do not use lubricants or saliva.* The list ended there, leaving the reader to use her imagination to cover the skipped steps. *Stroke penis with designated hand only, holding the sterile container firmly in the other, non-moving hand. Form secure grip on penis by overlapping thumb and index finger. Try to avoid contact with testicles for sanitary reasons. Remember to remove all non-sterile rings, watches, buttons, zippers, etc. If hand brushes penis tip, swab with unused medi-wipe and begin again at step four (stroke penis, etc. . . .).*

Sure, we'd joked about this day, the cold, clinical room, that single chair you just knew had been masturbated in countless times by hopeful dad after hopeful donor, the simulated-leather lounger most likely purchased from a superstore that could have ended up anywhere—at a student lounge, in a coffee shop—but is here instead. We thought perhaps if you listened very carefully, you might be able to hear it scream every time a new guy walked in. If viewed with a black light, would the room appear bespattered as a Jackson Pollock? Some officious nurse would hand Gary a stack of ragged, aged porn magazines and expect him to perform as the sound of everyday clinic doings penetrated the door. But I knew that the strict instructions for carrying out something that had previously been done at will and for selfish pleasure, combined with a small, plastic, sharp-lipped vagina dentata of a sterile cup, was no laughing matter.

"Honey?" Gary asks, watching the traffic behind us in his rearview mirror. "I don't want you to take this the wrong way. But what's our current policy on adoption? I mean, at what point do we throw in the biological towel?"

"Jesus, Gary. We haven't even failed yet, and you're already making backup plans. That's fucking great."

"It's my nature. I think it behooves us to establish a contingency plan. You know, for our peace of mind."

"It'd jinx us to talk about it. Let's hold off."

"*Au contraire,*" he says. "It'd jinx us not to have a Plan B. I say we do this twice, and if it doesn't happen by then, let's call it quits."

"What happens if I get pregnant but miscarry? Does that count as 'not happening'? What if I don't get pregnant either time, but Dr. Hamlin assures us three's the charm? Do we walk away from all this medical expertise and cutting-edge technology based purely on some oral agreement made under duress and out of ignorance?"

"I suppose," Gary says. "But don't say I didn't warn you."

Of all the issues Gary and I had dealt with during the six years we'd been together, the small disagreements over prosaic happenings were nothing compared to the stress of IVF. In fact, nothing had prepared us, as a couple or as individuals, for it.

According to Alice Domar of Boston IVF's Mind/Body Center, infertility is often the first major crisis a couple faces, the first real time one half of a couple must confront the way the other, possibly romanticized half endures and deals with catastrophe. Men and women typically react differently, explains Domar. Most of her women patients not only feel more depressed than their male partners, but are also raring to pursue aggressive treatments sooner.

"I'd say very few of the couples I've seen have been in the same place at the same time," she says. "They seem to be on different planets, with the woman often ahead by about a year. Often she's upset that he isn't more upset, and he's upset that she's so upset. She typically feels that he's holding her back; he typically feels that she's pushing him into decisions."

Despite the fact that 17 percent of couples of childbearing age experience infertility troubles, I couldn't help but believe that out of all the men sitting in Hamlin's waiting room, mine seemed the most skeptical, and the illest prepared.

I had listened to Cara Alberts when she explained that partners who agree strongly on how to deal with stressful life events can successfully manage their impact. I had paid attention. But with all of our bickering and the fact I was way more eager to hit the hard stuff as often as required to yield that genetic child, I started to fear that Gary and I might not weather this crisis, which wouldn't be that big a tragedy, really, since there'd be no kids involved, no visitation to work out, no custody battles. But if I had a baby, the ultimate disaster would be averted and all would be well, a totally asinine belief in using a positive result to bandage a festering wound.

Carol had assured me that most people find aspiration "not unpleasant. A slight prick. Like a bee sting. That is, under adequate sedation."

"What would it feel like without the anesthesia?" I wondered.

"I have an idea," Carol said. "Why don't you try it and report back? It'd be good practice for a natural childbirth, if that's also something you're curious about. If you get pregnant, that is."

"I was just asking," I said, clarifying that my preprocedure paperwork reflected my strong preference for being put under. Great Lakes called it a "twilight sedation," because you're not completely asleep but rather in a sort of la-la state in which you feel no pain and remember no offense. Even had I not known the meaning, I still would have liked the sound of it, like they'd be getting me high at sunrise or sunset, granting me sweet relief not only from the ache of the hollow needle suctioning eggs from my tender ovaries but from the emotional intensity of the past month. I'd be blissed out, floating in my own world. It sounded like absolute heaven.

"You sure that's a good idea?" Gary asks on the drive up when I remind him about the sedation.

"Why not?"

"Because you might end up pregnant in a couple days, that's why not. You've begun taking prenatal vitamins, you stopped using saccharin. If you're already working on the kid's digs, I'd think narcotics would top the Prohibited list."

"If it wasn't safe for the fetus, they wouldn't offer it," I say.

"Embryo. Didn't you learn this in junior high? Haven't the nurses been talking about it? Good Lord, haven't you been reading the materials provided? It's not a fetus right off the bat. It's an embryo."

"Fetus. Embryo. You know what I mean. And anyway, the embryo doesn't have a brain that drugs can negatively impact. So yeah, I think I do mean fetus."

"All I know is," Gary says, "I'm starving to death." I haven't been allowed to eat, so he decided to abstain from breakfast as a show of support.

"Hey, no big deal," he said when I thanked him for the team spirit. "It's going to be my kid, too. Only thing is, we'll likely hit rush-hour traffic. Maybe I should pack a yogurt or a starchy carb so I won't feel nauseous in the operating room."

"As I told you, Gary, I don't care if you eat. I hate merely symbolic gestures, although I will accept flowers on Mother's Day if this works."

"No, no. You're right. I should stick to my guns. I'm fasting. With you. Because I want to share in your physical discomfort. From now until we get back home, consider me on a hunger strike."

We pull into the parking lot of Great Lakes Fertility with time to spare. "See that one really tall evergreen?" Gary asks. He swerves into the loading area in front of the squat office building belonging to Highland Park Hospital. "I grew up about two miles west of it. I kind of like that our kids might come into being so close to where I lived. And they'll be born east of the Edens, in the fancy section of town. It's the American dream, all right."

"Do you really think this is when they're born? At the moment of creation?" Suddenly I feel sick to my stomach. This is such a profound idea. Also, my socially liberal husband sounds so right-wing. "God, this is the moment of creation, isn't it? When your sperm hits my egg and the nuclei react. I mean, really, life does begin at this cellular level. And some anonymous professional type will be the one who pulls the trigger on this thing that might end up being not only our kid but a person who will celebrate a lifetime of birthdays determined by the precise timing of a medical procedure and a stranger's technique."

"It's okay, hon. That's how this works. Hey, that's sort of how regular conception works. Now go inside and I'll park the car."

I lean over and kiss him. "Please hurry."

The waiting room is already full, but this time with almost equal numbers of men and women. I check in.

"Feinerman. First on the list. How'd you swing that?" asks an unfamiliar and upbeat woman sitting behind the reception desk. She is in full makeup, despite the hour, and her hair is in an elaborate up-do involving coiled braids and a fabric flower. "Go straight on back, take a right at the end of the hall, and look for Carol, who'll give you your gown and show you to your waiting area."

"My husband is parking the car," I say.

"Don't worry. I'll let him know where you are. They won't be ready for you until the other members of your batch show up anyway."

I walk through the swinging door and see that they've transformed the back into a makeshift triage unit, with portable, tented rooms like in an ER or the set of *M*A*S*H*. Carol waits at the end of the hall, watching me come toward her. She wears blue scrubs, and her clogged foot taps faster than I can walk.

"Showtime." I don't know what else to say. "I'm sort of nervous and excited. I hope it works, after everything."

"Of course you do," Carol says. "You're in room one. Remove all your clothes except your socks, if you wish. No contact lenses allowed. Do you have any loose teeth? Put this cap on and try to get all your hair inside. Where's your partner?"

"He's parking the car. He should be here any minute."

"Jeez. Okay. He's not allowed inside the operating room during aspiration anyway."

I find room one, slide the curtain closed, and undress. As I struggle to get the last of my hair inside the puffy disposable cap, a woman ducks her head inside my room. The same hat looks great on her—delicate and gauzy, the baby blue a perfect match for her eyes.

"Hi. I'm Debbie the embryologist. We spoke on the phone." She extends a hand. "Let's see here." She checks the file with the enormous 20125 sticker on it. "We should discuss your options." She glances around. "Where's your partner?"

"He should be here. He was parking the car." I hear Gary say my name. I hear Carol say, "Nice of you to show up. Room One."

"Here I am. Sorry," Gary says, excusing himself and squeezing by Debbie.

"Gary. This is the embryologist."

"Debbie," Debbie says, extending her hand toward Gary. They shake. He has powdered sugar on his thumb.

Debbie continues, "According to the results from your last ultrasound, you have about two dozen fairly large follicles. What would you like to do in case we're able to fertilize more than the amount we transfer back into your uterus, all things working out as we hope?"

"Why do we have to decide this now?" I ask. "Isn't it counting our chickens? Didn't somebody say you call after the retrieval to discuss options?"

"We like to get a firm read before aspiration. We've found that after fertilization emotion creeps in. People start identifying with the embryos, which muddies their judgment. Also, sometimes a woman has a sort of anesthesia hangover that might cause her to say something contrary to her true beliefs. And for legal reasons, we need to have your embryo dispensation forms on file before we even have embryos."

"What are the options?" asks Gary, focused as ever.

"Cryopreservation, donation, or discarding."

"Whoa," Gary says.

"Really? That's it?" I ask, surprised not to have been presented with this stuff before. "Why didn't we talk about this earlier?"

"Cryo. As in frozen?" Gary asks Debbie.

"Yes. We have a storage facility here. You'd share a tank with other families, but we mark all the straws clearly and bill you annually, which also works well as a reminder that the embryos still exist. You look confused. A *straw* is another term for the containers we freeze the embryos in. They look a lot like drinking straws."

"No," I say. "I was just wondering who could forget about their frozen embryos."

"You'd be surprised. Once people achieve a healthy live birth, particularly if it's a second or third child, they like to put this entire ordeal out of their minds, leftovers included."

"Not us," I say, suddenly confident. "We haven't discussed it yet, but I imagine we'd want to preserve our unused embryos. Try to defrost—is that what you'd call it?—and use them in the future. Right, Gary?" I ask, while going ahead and signing the paper clipped to the outside of the folder Debbie holds toward me. Gary says he guesses so, if that's what I want.

"Great," Debbie says. "Expect to hear from me first thing tomorrow morning with a report on how many eggs fertilized and how they're looking, as well as a recommendation for a three- or five-day transfer. Good luck." She shakes both our hands a final time, then scoots backward out of our chamber, slides the curtain closed, and introduces herself to the people in the next alcove.

"Frozen embryos," Gary says. "Man. I'll bet everybody makes the same jokes about that. You know, future ice skaters or baby Martha Stewarts, that kind of thing."

"Oh. Because she's cold. Right. Anyway, I think these tented rooms are called berths," I say, remembering this from a Word-A-Day Calendar I had in junior high. "With an *e*, not an *i*. Then again, I think that might somehow involve a ship."

"You ignoring me?" Gary asked.

"What do you mean?"

"Joking aside, do you suppose once-frozen kids incur any significant physical damage? The human equivalent of freezer burn?"

"How do I know? Man, I can't believe this is the first time the subject even came up. But even if we'd had time to think it through, don't think I'd let a little rime prevent me from using them. Any birth includes its fair share of risk, right? I mean, plenty of people use ultrasound or amniocentesis and end up finding out their baby has a problem but still proceed with the pregnancy."

"Yeah, but that's different. The baby is already in them, gestating and forming and developing. It has a heart and limbs and a brain. Frozen embryos are a totally separate category. Potential potential life as opposed to actual potential life."

"You're splitting hairs," I say. "And anyway, I don't want to make a decision that forecloses all others, particularly since I have no idea how I'll feel once I know all the facts. I don't see how there's any choice but to freeze them now and figure it out later."

Gary looks at me and shakes his head. "Fine. It's your call. But don't let this turn you into a monster."

"Meaning?"

"Okay. Well, let's say we have a kid or two without ever having to tap into the frozen supply. We're satisfied and love our kids and raise them, and they move out and we grow old."

"Ooh. Scary."

"So we're old, right? But we still have these embryos. I can see us sitting on our rocking chairs, sipping Tummy Wellness tea, the sun glinting off my bald head, lint accumulating in your crow's-feet. We're bored, lonely, retired. We remember, despite our flagging mental agility, the frozen embryos and decide, what the Sam Hill, let's go for it. We take the retirement home shuttle to Highland Park Hospital, and I totter to the reception desk and start banging on it with my cane until somebody appears. It's Dr. Hamlin! He still looks great! Tan and trim as ever, thanks to his access to all the latest medical advancements.

"'I'm here for my kids,' I'll demand. 'Now goddammit, we've waited fifty years, paid our annual storage fee that, with inflation, brings us to fifty thousand simoleons. But you remember Beth. No? Well, when she makes up her mind, there's no stopping her. She's feeling maternal, gramaternal, really, and nothing you say is going to stop us.'

"And then you know what Dr. Hamlin says? He tells us no problem, since he's worked with us before and all. So we have a baby in our seventies, and you feel vital again. Not young, exactly, but youthful. Technically enabled or not, the life-force is still the life-force. And we don't even care so much that our kid is stuck with these literally lame, pathetic, hubristic parents or that we'll have to convert a corner of our assisted-living apartment into a nursery. I guess my point is that we should always remember that capability and appropriateness are very different things, and even if we can span the gap with technology, that's a very slippery bridge indeed."

"Thank you, Dr. Leon Kass," I say. I compliment Gary on his imagination and the amusing bit of science fiction to brighten up an otherwise overwhelming morning. But saving our embryos for future use, or not, is a grave decision, one with massive moral implications. We need time to think about it, explore our feelings around having a huge family, destroying the leftovers, or donating them to science or another couple. And if we decide to use them, how can that be accomplished in a moral way? If we thaw them all out and use only one, won't that be 99 percent as offensive as destroying them in the first place? What is the alternative? To de-ice one or two and keep the rest stranded, or be faced with the same dilemma farther down the road but this time with even more Feinerman children tugging at our practical sides? Alas, we need to decide on the spot. So we sign the cryopreservation sheet simply because it is the only choice that won't foreclose all others.

After about an hour in the tented room, a period I spend listening to fellow patients talking with their escorts, Carol fetches me. Gary kisses me goodbye. I tell him I love him and that I'll be fine, wish him luck with the specimen, wince a little to let him know I am down with his potential discomfort, and follow Carol to the procedure room. Masked and bootied people perform various jobs. I try to hoist myself onto the gynecological chair without exposing myself to the assemblage.

"Which arm has the bigger veins?" Carol asks.

"My left one. But that's where most of my blood tests have been. It might be cashed by now."

Carol examines the crook in my left arm, bending and straightening it. Bend. Straighten. "This'll do," she says. She slaps at the veins a few times, then plants the IV anesthetic needle. "This is the twilight drip. It'll put you mostly to sleep. Try not to talk. It's hard to make sense when you're on this, and you'll most likely regret whatever you manage."

When I wake up, Dr. Hamlin is sitting across from me, the foot crossed over his knee slowly circling. "St. Croix," he seems to say.

"St. Croix?" I hear myself mumble. "I've never been to St. Croix. What about St. Croix?" I turn my head and spot Gary. *What are you laughing at, sexy man?*

"You've been inquiring after my tan. I was telling you about my trip to St. Croix. It looks like you're waking up, Liz." He calls me Liz. I've clarified that it is Elizabeth or Beth, never Liz. Not that Liz isn't a perfectly nice name—it just isn't mine. "Before our chat about the islands, I was informing Gary that the procedure went superbly. I was able to gather twenty nice-sized follicles. I'm quite pleased."

"Good. I'm so glad," I say. "Hey, Dr. Hamlin. Where'd you get that great tan?"

Gary walks slowly with me, carrying my purse, to the waiting area just inside the electronic front doors and tells me to have a seat, he'll get the car. The doors whoosh noisily as he breezes through them and jogs into the parking lot. Woozy from the anesthesia, I fear I'll throw up right there in the pristine lobby, next to the Naugahyde benches and beneath the giant prints of Picasso's *Guernica*. My pelvis feels like it weighs a ton, heavier even than before they removed the dozen and a half eggs. What if they've left a piece of equipment behind, like those surgical sponges that sometimes turn up encased, and festering, in postoperative abdomens, that they'll rediscover on whichever day I come back for my embryo transfer? What if my body and mind are so primed for pregnancy that whatever Hamlin has left inside me takes up residence and starts to ripen? I'll go into a state of hysterical pregnancy, and when the obstetrician fails to detect a heartbeat, I'll mourn the loss of my child, even if it had only ever been a torn piece of latex or plastic catheter part.

Feverishly, I manage to hoist myself out of the seat and into the fresh air. I spot our old Volvo coming toward me (looking way too much like something parents drive and how dare we presume?). Gary, on the inside, is yelling words I can't hear. He beeps the horn and flashes the lights, a vehicular scolding for having gotten up. An elderly lady in a gigantic sedan turns in front of Gary, cutting him off. I sit down on the sidewalk. Several people ask if I'm okay, and I tell every last one of them, "Not really."

As we ride home, I ask Gary to keep the radio off and the windows rolled down. Reclining in the passenger seat, I listen to cars whiz by and semis head in the other direction. I watch treetops, tall buildings, overpasses roll by. A kid on an overpass waves. As we near him, he looks down through my window, smiles, and waves his gloved hand a little faster. There's my omen. He is there for me, a beacon of hope whose parents should know better than to let him out alone where he might take up position by the expressway to wave to strangers, some of whom may not have my awesome regard for children, and for the careless parents blessed enough to have them.

The next morning all I can think about is Debbie's call. At 11:00 a.m., three hours after I'd started expecting it, the phone rings.

"Is this Liz? It's Debbie from the lab. We've successfully fertilized nineteen eggs. I checked with Dr. H. this morning, and at this point we're both recommending blastocyst."

I'm impatient, a control freak, traits I've had to quash for the past month. I ache to reclaim what's rightfully mine. My embryos. My reproductive capabilities. Mine, mine, mine. I'm a mother bird forced off her nest in desperate, visceral need of an immediate reunion. I lower my voice, even though Gary's not home, and demur.

"We'd prefer a three-day transfer. I mean, ultimately it is our choice, correct?"

"You just need to know how risky that'd be. If I were the gambling type, which the folks at Harrah's Hollywood Casino keep telling me I am, I'd put a chunk of change on multiples. These are strong embryos, and you're on the young side."

"We don't mind assuming that risk. We're not talking about replacing more than three, right?"

"But if you wait until day five, we'll only transfer two proven embryos. And you could still very well end up with twins."

"Debbie, I know you're the pro, but enough playing God. We've spent the last month pulling strings meant to be invisible and ethereal. We've taken all the wonder, the nature, the mystery out of having a kid, from the handpicked sperm to the manufactured eggs, injecting the sperm directly inside to nicking the eggshell to encourage growth. I mean, I can't take any further loss of romance. Would it be so wrong to back off a little from the technology, place these embryos in their natural environment where they belong, and let nature take over?"

"Well, we do keep the embryos at optimal conditions. The stage of the microscope, where the embryos are placed, is heated to exactly thirty-seven degrees Celsius, which is body temperature. And microscopes don't have fevers or viruses or any of the problems that people have. We have far greater control with embryos kept outside the body. Of course it's not my decision, but you're drawing an arbitrary line. Remember, in vitro fertilization literally means "fertilization in glass." Glass. Not tissue, not carnal, but glass, of the petri dish or test tube variety. You knew what this would entail, and frankly I'm surprised you'd retreat from the best science has to offer and resort to finger-crossing." Debbie sighs and clears her throat. "I suppose the worst that could happen is you end up with trips. Unless, of course, one of the three embryos spontaneously divides. But like I said, worse things have happened."

"Yeah," I say. "Worse, as in, having gone through all this and not getting pregnant. Or, how about if we waited for blastocyst, and between tomorrow and Friday Highland Park Hospital floods or explodes or gets in the path of a tornado? What if I have a catastrophic car accident on Friday morning? If I'm choosing, I'm choosing pregnancy enough for three people rather than none at all."

I phone Gary and tell him the great news about how many fertilized embryos we have and that he'll need to take Friday off since we'll be going in for a three-day transfer.

"No way. We're doing blastocyst," he says, knocking my socks off with the fact that he's been paying attention.

"What do you know about it?" I ask.

"After I finished producing the specimen and while you were still recovering, I looked through some literature and talked to Debbie about the pros and cons of blastocyst. As far as I can tell, and in her expert opinion, there really is no choice. Blastocyst is the state of the art and the way to prevent putting in embryos that won't thrive at days four and five as well as to avoid having twins or triplets."

"I'd love to have twins or triplets—get the whole thing over with at once."

"I'm not sure I'll have enough in me to parent one kid, let alone two or three. I've let you call all the shots up until now. I was against freezing, if you want to know the truth. Get pregnant, and you're back in the driver's seat. But this time I'm siding with the experts. I love you, but you're out of your depth."

I call Great Lakes and notify them as to our change of plans.

8

Almonds,
Watermelons,
and Pears

Like most of the things I've neglected throughout my life—
my car's brake pads, the expiration date stamped on hummus
containers, a childhood gerbil named Happy who disappeared
from his cage unnoticed, turning up dead months later at the
back of my closet—I didn't concern myself with my reproductive health until the rattling and fuzz and stiffening had already
set in. How stupid I'd been to assume my machinery well oiled,
my raw materials fresh and functional, this when a package of
Tampax purchased in the late 1980s sat unopened, perched on
a bathroom shelf, a light layer of dust coating its seafoam-green
top.

It mattered little that I was already thirty when I decided to
have a baby—my PCO made the age factor a moot one. But it
bothered me, made me feel the ignoramus for having assumed
all was well, despite the indications to the contrary, and despite
the pragmatic filter through which I customarily view the
world and my shaky place in it.

Normally, I expend gobs of mental energy worrying about a multitude of potential health crises: my heart petering out while I sleep, blood clots silently creeping along my venous system on their way to permanent, and devastating, lodging in my lungs and/or brain, food poisoning, antibiotic resistance, degenerative eye problems, loud-music-induced hearing loss, raw-food-induced parasites, hormones in my chicken, worms in my pork. So where was my customary prophylactic alarm—that superstitious deflection of the evil eye—when it came to this most precarious and invisible of physical structures, my re-productive system?

I'd started taking birth control pills in college, not only to prevent an unwanted pregnancy but also to mark a colossal milestone: the inception of my sex life. It's what mature, college-age women did, I figured. It was what all my friends were doing. We had intercourse, mostly with boyfriends, but first we took precautions to prevent unwelcome outcomes—pregnancy, the clap, AIDS.

For this reason, and because I believed that eighteen years of near absolute purity and all that high school abstinence had rendered me, and my various virgin regions, superfertile, I in-sisted that my boyfriend and I double up on the birth control, using a pill-condom combo. I also insisted he get a blood test to confirm that he was negative for HIV and STD-free. The way I saw it, all my former seclusion from the male world had impacted my ova, turning them into desperados, like a bunch of lonely men in lockdown, up for any sexual encounter, no matter the quality or quantity. It'd work like homeopathy: the slightest vestige of sperm, one millionth of a part even, would reach my ripening egg, and next thing I knew, I'd be having a tearful discussion with a guy who was supposed to mean little in the long run.

So I took oral contraceptives methodically, year after year, a decade's worth, until I met and married Gary, saw Dr. Frank-furth, and found out there hadn't been much chance I'd needed them at all. They'd been a redundancy, efficacious as a sugar pill, like an Ambien regimen for Rip Van Winkle, or Spanish fly sprinkled atop Mary Kay Letourneau's Malt-O-Meal.

Still, it felt good, satisfying even, to pop the small tablets lined up in their perfect rows of seven through the back of the foil sheet, leaving tiny and almost identical tears and neat lines of emptied pods, like shell casings or a parking lot filled with abandoned spacecraft, as, day by day and dose by dose, I closed in on that fourth row of dummy pills thoughtfully included to help us ladies sustain our birth control routines, even as we endured a week of bleeding, bloating, and cramping and the less tidy feminine-specific items we'd have no choice but to enlist.

The birth control pill manufacturers did a good job of creating packaging that resembled something thunk up by Mattel. Pearlescent pink, trim and discreet, each prescription included a plastic compact within which to tuck one's monthly supply. It's what Barbie would take if ovaries and oocytes lurked within her pinched waist and if Ken had the cojones. In recent years the packaging has evolved, the rectangular compacts mostly giving way to mod-looking round dispensers, the pills circling round the center. Then there's Yasmin, the oral contraceptive I'm now on (to keep my hormones balanced and my complexion blemish-free), which comes with a jewel-tone, sueded moleskin wallet, looking like something the *Queer Eye* guys would choose for Davy Crockett.

Ovaries are a woman's primary reproductive organs and the warehouse for her lifetime supply of eggs. Almondish in both shape and size, they are situated in the ovarian fossae, shallow depressions on either side of the uterus in the lateral walls of the pelvic cavity and held loosely in place by peritoneal ligaments. Male bodies, under normal conditions, produce sperm throughout their life spans, but a woman's ovaries contain all the oocytes (female germ cells within the follicles that, when exposed to hormones at puberty, develop into eggs) she will ever have or, if nothing goes wrong, need. When a girl is born, she carries into the world her roughly 700,000 oocytes, which, like a new car driven off the showroom floor, begin their decline the moment they take up position in the flow of human traffic. By puberty, the number will have decreased to around 400,000.

Many of ART's best customers have egg-quality issues. Mostly they're older women who put off childbearing for one reason or another—education, career, lack of a suitable partner, fear of taking care of a child, doubts over their body's ability to produce a healthy one, total faith in their body and/or medicine to achieve pregnancy on demand, and a ton of other good reasons—and need fertility drugs either to tweak their own eggs or to acquire some from donors.

Sylvia Ann Hewlett, economist and director of the Gender and Public Policy Program at Columbia's School of International and Public Affairs, in her 2002 book *Creating a Life: Professional Women and the Quest for Children*, examined the population of successful women who postponed reproduction until their careers were well established, only to discover they'd waited too long. She found that, by the age of forty, between a third and a half were childless, but only 14 percent had planned it that way. Hewlett writes, "Feminism and the pill have given women more choices, but cannot change medical realities. Few women over the age of 40 will be able to conceive and bear children easily." She offers only one solution: for young women to reorder their priorities if it's biological offspring they're after.

The promise that IVF holds for overcoming biological limitations, and the real-life examples of older mommies pushing twins and triplets around the streets we live on, lead many women to assume they'll be able to have kids some way, somehow. But the truth is, if it's a 100 percent biologically related child they want, even IVF can't help most women over forty. Using donor eggs or gestational surrogates is a wonderful solution, but the question has increasingly become whether to impose a cutoff age for becoming a parent.

A recent CDC report, issued in January 2005, shows that the younger a woman is when she uses ART, the more likely she is to become pregnant using her own eggs and end up with a live birth. Thirty-seven percent of women who undergo ART using their own fresh eggs when they're 35 or younger successfully give birth. But only 31 percent of women between 35 and 37 do so; 21 percent of women between 38 and 40; 11 percent of women between 41 and 42; and just 4 percent of women over 42. However, using donated eggs neutralizes the woman's age as a factor. In 2002 the live birth rate for all ART procedures using donor eggs was 50 percent, and the success rate varied only slightly among age groups.

Victoria Wright, one of the CDC report's authors, summed up the data: "Women in their twenties and early thirties who used ART had the most success with pregnancies and single live births . . . success rates declined steadily once a woman reached her mid-thirties." The figures, she added, should act as "a reminder that age remains a primary factor with respect to pregnancy success, and younger women have greater success than older women, even with technology."

In 1997 a sixty-three-year-old California woman, married to her sixty-year-old husband for sixteen years without any other children, became the oldest birth mother on record in the United States when she had a (perfectly healthy) baby girl. Since then around a thousand women in their fifties and sixties have given birth in America. A sixty-six-year-old Romanian had a baby in 2003, as did a sixty-five-year-old Indian in 2005.

The Californian underwent IVF at the University of Southern California School of Medicine, using a donor egg and her husband's sperm. When she first presented herself at the clinic, she claimed to be fifty years old. Only after she'd com-

pleted her first trimester did she level with her obstetrician, letting him know she was in her sixties and therefore too old to
have qualified for USC's treatment program, which like many
clinics has an age limit of fifty-five.

Her fertility doctor, Richard Paulson, director of USC Fertility, said that even though a decade of research had proven
that implantation and full-term pregnancy can occur no matter a woman's age, he would not have accepted her into the
program had he known she was over fifty-five. But he also
made clear that this patient passed the screening tests and produced multiple medical records, all confirming she was fifty-
three at the time of IVF. "We had no reason to doubt her word,
and we were not trying to set any records. The average age of
women coming to us for oocyte donation is forty-three." Of her
conception and healthy pregnancy, he said, "It may be that
women have not one but two biological clocks—the clock for
the eggs and ovaries seems to run out much earlier than the
one for the uterus."

Interviewed on PBS's *NewsHour*, Dr. Paulson explained
USC's rationale for choosing fifty-five, an age at which a woman
is "pushing the limit" for a safe, healthy pregnancy. For one
thing, fifty-five is a nice, round number and close enough to
the average age of natural menopause (fifty-one) to not seem
too aggressive, yet still around ten years past the age at which
natural child-bearing normally ends, giving the medical advances room to do what it is they do. Most women at forty-five,
even though they are commonly still cycling normally, are
highly unlikely to become pregnant without egg donation. So
fifty-five is kind of an arbitrary extension of nature by about ten
years, long enough to give the medicine a chance but still
within the limits of medical responsibility and social acceptance.

When the California woman gave birth, the reaction was
fervent and mixed. A sixty-plus mother just plain gave some
people the heebie-jeebies. Here was this postmenopausal

woman tinkering with Mother Nature, forcing an innocent fetus to gestate in decrepit digs and condemning her to the stigma of having an Old Lady Mom. Some people, not knowing the patient had misled the clinic, considered USC's willingness to work with a woman in her sixties unabashedly mercenary, using it to prove the unethical potentials of reproductive manipulation. A grandmother-aged first-time mother was only the beginning, they claimed; the cloning of human beings and the use of large, nonhuman mammals—cows and dromedaries—as gestational surrogates was surely close behind, options that would be made available according to customer demand and ability to pay.

But in a society that values (or merely tolerates, or looks for chances to rein in) the right of women to make reproductive choices for themselves, the medical establishment has difficulty instituting consistent policy for determining who should or should not attempt parenthood. Perhaps the fulfillment of certain health criteria should be the sole determinant. So, if a would-be mother, no matter her age, has a primo electrocardiogram, clear, elegant fallopian tubes, and original uterus intact, passes a stress test, is of sound mind, regularly exercised and healthily fed body—in other words, if her slightly wrinkled skin glows with good health and a mothering sort of warmth—how could the docs claim she is a worse candidate than the overweight, diabetic twenty-eight-year-old wearing a T-shirt with the words "Shut Up" in rhinestone lettering, noshing on Ding-Dongs as she fills out her clinical paperwork using a cigarette-shaped pen?

Most doctors agree that in determining how old is too old, the safety of the mother is the principal consideration. "We know that the mother is at increased risk for any number of other medical complications even, say, at the age of forty as compared with thirty. And if you extrapolate from that on to beyond fifty and so forth, it is likely that this risk will increase.

How much that risk increases we just don't know," Dr. Paulson explains.

One concern is that with advancing age, uterine blood vessels may not be able to adapt to pregnancy, when the uterus grows from the size of a pear to that of a watermelon. Another concern is that age may predispose women to certain pregnancy complications, such as diabetes, blood clots in the legs, or cardiovascular strain, since during pregnancy the heart works that much harder, pumping blood to nourish both the maternal body and the placenta. The older a birth mother gets, the greater the risk of premature birth and birth defect. But putting aside the physically fit California applicant who fudged her birth date on every last form, the demand for fertility services beyond the age of fifty is not high, and upward of sixty almost nonexistent.

A July 2005 story on NPR's *All Things Considered* looked at two fertility clinics grappling with the age issue. Dr. Elizabeth Ginsburg, medical director of the ART program at Boston's Brigham and Women's Hospital, drew an important distinction between being biologically too old to bear a child and being vital enough to raise a child one neither bore nor contributed an egg toward. The question in the latter case really becomes whether people are too old to parent, at some point, and whether the medical establishment should be deciding that issue.

Recently two women in their fifties came to Brigham and Women's Hospital, seeking help in conceiving a child. Both women planned on using donor eggs and gestational surrogates, but the hospital ethics committee had to decide whether to work with them, even if they had no biological involvement in the pregnancy. Dr. Ginsburg explains that the clinicians weren't comfortable proclaiming who is and is not allowed to raise a child. "So it's something we really triaged to our own internal ethics committee, which consists of people in the health care area in our field. We really couldn't reach a consensus and then brought it to the hospital ethics committee, which is a much broader base of the health care system and also involves women and men from the community. So we felt that it would be a better representation of what society's feeling was."

Arguments against a cutoff age included the fact that there exists no cutoff for men, which struck some committee members as unfair and outright discriminatory, despite the natural and common condition of sperm viability even into a man's twilight years. Concerns also centered on the potential for a child to be orphaned at a young age, even though gerontologists taking part in the discussions debunked that idea. A healthy fifty-year-old woman, they said, will most likely still be alive and kicking at eighty. Committee members who favored a cutoff age for women felt it is selfish for a woman in her fifties to mother a child and that older parents are not in the best interest of the child. They ticked off proofs of this selfishness, such as the burden of caring for older parents and even the stigma of being known to have older parents.

These issues are new, and therefore no standard of care yet exists. Dr. Ginsburg surveyed colleagues around the country, looking for standards, and found a few different methods for imposing cutoffs. Some clinics use composite age as the qualifying factor, with one hundred as the most commonly used number. So if the combined age of the couple is one hundred or less, technically they'll be given the green light, no matter the span between the two integers, the elder's gender, or the social issues suggested by the eighty-year-old geezer husband and his twenty-year-old wife or vice versa. Others, like Brigham and Women's and USC, use fifty-five as the cutoff age. They admit it's an arbitrary number, but when forced to make arbitrary decisions, to establish policy where none came before, one does so in a way that makes some intuitive sense, that feels comfortable and medically responsible, but that still allows room for the medical breakthroughs to blossom.

NPR also interviewed Dr. Robert Stillman of the Shady Grove Fertility Center in Rockville, Maryland, who argues that fixing an uppermost age limit on medically assisted conception is an easy call. Principally, a cutoff should be placed where medical therapies cease to succeed. Shady Grove, therefore, does not offer IVF to women over forty-four because, quite simply, that's the age when most women's eggs cease to be viable. Women over fifty-one cannot undergo IVF using donor eggs at Shady Grove, because fifty-one is the average age for onset of menopause. Biology guides Dr. Stillman, who explains, "Most physicians are not interested in extending the reproductive life span, whether that be earlier than puberty— because we can induce ovulation in an eight-year-old, but no one would ever consider doing that, hopefully. And menopausal women after their reproductive life has ended would not come under medical therapy, either."

Implicit in this biological standard is a recognition that people age at different rates, some remaining healthy and vital, physically fit, and mentally sharp even while their contemporaries slow down, stoop, and lose orientation. So for them the menopause measure makes sense. It not only addresses the unfairness that comes with choosing patients on a case-by-case basis, but also is directly related to reproductive age, having nothing to do with a potential patient's tennis acumen or transcendent yoga poses, her finesse as a surgeon, or her success as a baker. Rather, nature's time line provides the perfect, logical, and natural gauge for determining when one's offspring-having days are over. A doctor's charge is to treat patients. It is his honor and his duty to do so. But a patient can be defined only as an individual with a medical disorder. Menopause is not a medically defined disorder, and therefore the menopausal woman is within neither the duty nor the purview of a medical doctor to treat. Case closed.

Perhaps my prime candidacy for IVF is what enabled me to take it relatively in stride, blindly following each day's instructions as they came, not worrying too terribly if I fumbled one small step or another. I was eligible for IVF by every measure: age, general health, insurance. My tubes were unobstructed. I had a uterus. All systems go.

Of course, I was consumed with fear about its aftereffects: that it might not work, that I'd never be pregnant or give birth. I also worried about the physical discomfort, indignities, and disappointments that surely awaited me, and I loathed, loathed, loathed my body for its epic failure. But more to the point, I was pissed at myself, the brain and guts part of myself, for not realizing somehow that something was amiss. I was embarrassed by my naïve prelapsarian self.

As for my eggs, it wasn't until I first saw their image on the ultrasound monitor that I fully appreciated them. They started off as tiny specks (and a ton of them, polycystic as I am), like buckshot or birdseed. Then as the cycle progressed and the medicine took effect, a smaller number of growing follicles emerged, responding to the drugs in the exact way Dr. Hamlin had described. It made me feel normal. Like despite the polycystic disorder, my body was still capable of functioning properly, albeit in a medically directed way. I began looking forward to that part of my appointments, the chance to peek inside my body and gauge the medical impact—so dramatic, so quick—and to watch the beginnings of what might, a little over nine months hence, be the baby I transport home from the hospital.

With my new appreciation and enthusiasm for my eggs, and a Pollyanna-ish distortion caused by the nostalgic glow of retrospect, the ova began to occupy my thoughts, more precious than anything cooked up by Fabergé. I scrolled back in time, trying to visualize them at various points in my life. What had their overall quality been while I was taking my SATs? Had the bass beat of Duran Duran at the prom reached their inner sanctum, the boom boom effecting little hiccups in my ovaries like reproductive maracas? They'd endured nights of

drinking, countless Grateful Dead concerts, bad job interviews, even worse jobs, good and bad boyfriends, a serious
courtship, and a really serious African honeymoon with a
newly married Gary and me.

My eggs had been there since my eighteenth gestational
week, quietly occupying their tiny portion of my body. Unlike
the showoff parts, the tongue and the biceps, the growling
stomach and ringing eardrums, the aching tooth and the
purple-blue threads on the inner wrists like anatomical embroidery, the ova were patient and noiseless. I pictured them
in the ovaries, these perfectly elliptical morsels, glowing with
a hidden backlight (tucked behind the fallopian tubes, no
doubt), little bundles of eggs pristine enough to serve a tsar.

The nineteen ova that had responded to medication, grown
as hoped for, and been suctioned from their follicles were now
on their own, fertilized embryos attempting their continual
development those twenty miles north on I-94. As I waited the
five days for them to reach the blastocyst stage, I worried. Anything could happen to them, particularly since they had no
armor, no protection from the outside world, and were as vulnerable as newborn turtles scrambling from beach to sea,
mostly not surviving, being eaten by predators or toppled and
drowned by the surf. More vulnerable, really, shell-less as they
were.

If the petri dish got too warm or too cool, they were sunk. If
they were jostled or accidentally spit on or doused with glass
cleaner or any of the other things that I imagined could happen quite by mistake yet with devastating results, I'd never
forgive myself for abandoning them there. But I was just
following protocol, I told myself. No parent-donor patients allowed in the lab. And even if I could somehow prevail upon
Hamlin to let me stay and stand guard over them, I'd have only
myself to blame if something happened on my watch, if they
spontaneously ceased developing, say, or if I knocked the dish
over by mistake and it crashed to the floor and I couldn't find

the embryos and then I'd have to live my life knowing they'd been mopped up rather than placed inside me and it was entirely my fault.

The night before my embryo transfer, Carol phones to remind us we'll need to be at Great Lakes no later than six the following morning. "Don't be late," she admonishes. "The schedule is delicate. If you miss your spot, it's nearly impossible for us to shuffle you guys around."

"Who guys?" I ask. "Us or everybody?"

"What?"

"Are you talking about rearranging me and my husband, because we'd be really flexible."

"No," Carol says, "I was referring to all of you with fertilized embryos to transfer. By this time in a batch, our numbers naturally dwindle. But still there are seventeen procedures scheduled for tomorrow morning, each with a designated time slot based on individual circumstances and needs. If you're late and we stand around waiting until you're ready, it gets chaotic. And again, we can't just jump around at random—the lab has the embryos queued up."

"We'll be on time, not to worry. I just wondered what you meant, is all. So, we're first. Is that significant? Is our case less complicated, a cinch? Or maybe you put the hard cases first, when Hamlin is still fresh and you have all morning to tackle the big problems."

"Putting embryos back in is usually a straightforward procedure. Pretty quick and easy. I guess you just got lucky. Or unlucky, depending on how you see it. Again, six a.m. Do not, I repeat, do not be late. Please."

The truth is, I'm terrified we'll oversleep or hit traffic or suffer car problems, and I've even begun having that dream where you walk into a seminar hall, only to find the rest of your class—the ones who'd paid scant attention, who'd sat in the back few rows dozing or daydreaming or ridiculing the damp, drooping ovals of the professor's pitted-out shirt while you sat in front, taking freakishly detailed notes and raising your hand to ask the many questions that occurred to you, that's how hard you were listening—knee deep in the final exam you are now destined to fail.

I also continue to fret about our embryos being at Great Lakes, alone—that is, without us—and the sooner we are re-united, the better. Although we didn't technically create them, we are family and the only ones who really and truly care about their outcome, after the cellular stage, that is. It just feels so wrong, like we are irresponsible or uncaring or lack a certain instinct not to abandon our progeny.

I worry about arriving late, fighting to find a parking spot, running in, and being rushed through. What if, in their haste, they misplace our embryos? Or what if they load up the wrong ones—the Singhs' or the Camarettis'—and I carry somebody else's baby, suffer through someone else's labor, and nurse and fall in love with their beautiful child? And then they force me to give it back?

After not really sleeping all night, we get out of bed at the agreed-upon time (four a.m.), shower, and dress: me in my lucky socks and sweats with a loose enough drawstring waist-band not to squish my return-trip belly, Gary in a flannel hik-ing shirt, more outdoor gear for our intensely indoor pursuit. We hurry out to our car, noting the unusually balmy weather for Chicago in the winter. A thin layer of snow lines the tree limbs and blankets the yews, the white glowing in the darkness. The garage door creaks as Gary pushes it open, the door bang-ing into the car I parked too far forward. A neighbor's dog be-gins to bark.

I glance around our garage, at the single bare bulb sur-rounded by a tangle of wires and cobwebs, the shovels and ice picks leaning unsteadily against the wall, the giant rake with most of its teeth broken off. Ice skates with rusted blades dangle from the industrial shelving I've crashed into so many times that it threatens to topple onto the hood of our car. If we are to become parents, we'll need to take a good, hard look around and address the suddenly evident dangers all around us.

As we settle into the car and fasten our seat belts, I grab Gary's arm. Doesn't he think our chances are really very good? The way Dr. Hamlin gushes about the medical advances, the embryologist's extreme skill and Great Lakes' unparalleled lab, my advantageous age and superb egg quality, and Gary's not-too-negative sperm factor—of course it's going to work! The punctilious injection schedule! The specificity of the portion of my upper thigh to shoot—nine inches above the knee, two inches right of center! The practice stabbing a raw potato, and the way Carol complimented me on my precision and quickness—a Lupron sharpshooter, she'd said—of course, of course, of course!

"It might work," Gary says. "Dr. Hamlin seems to know what he's talking about. All set?"

"Yes," I say. "All set." We cruise west on Fullerton Parkway, catching mostly green lights. Everything is still closed, including the Dunkin' Donuts that I know Gary has pegged his wee-hour hopes upon.

We reach the on-ramp and merge with the already developing northbound traffic, listening to news of a suicide bombing on NPR. A delivery truck with "Fresh Appetizers by Chef Cesar" stenciled on the side catches up with us, and the driver looks in at me looking at him. He smiles and I smile back, and he zooms off, an action that leaves me suddenly and inexplicably aware that I am nervous about all the things that are out of my control this day. I am anxious about the profundity of the impending procedure and suddenly doubt whether Dr. Hamlin really knows what he is doing. I turn off the radio.

"Does Hamlin strike you as a little, I don't know, demented?"

"What are you talking about? I was listening to that."

"Just hear me out. Do you think Dr. Hamlin chose reproductive technology as his specialty mostly because it's way cooler than normal gynecological stuff? And the way he urged us to go directly to IVF, to not bother with insemination or any of the less complicated procedures. That's sort of mad scientist–ish, don't you think? And what about all those heliskiing magazines in his office? Do you think that's appropriate? If it were your waiting room, wouldn't you choose more general lifestyle magazines?"

"What would you prefer?" Gary asks. "*Parents Digest* or *Parade of Babies*? How about *Cosmo*, with all of those young, hot chicks with their flat bellies and uncomplicated sex lives? That'd be cruel." He reaches through the steering wheel and resets the odometer. "He likes skiing. Big deal—you like skiing. What, are you freaking out or something?"

"No, I'm just saying. I can't help but wonder whether Dr. Hamlin is in it 'cause it's daredevilish and pioneering. Like he wants to sink a tiny South African flag between the fimbriae of my fallopian tubes. And, of course, there are the medical journal write-ups . . ."

"It's just nerves and an attempt to protect yourself," Gary says. "You're using blame transference in case you don't get pregnant."

"Great diagnosis, Dr. Joyce Brothers. Perhaps if I had married the handsome daredevil scientist with the shiny Mercedes rather than an amateur psychologist wearing Grizzly Adams's threads we'd all be better off."

As soon as I finish, I feel terrible. This isn't easy for Gary, either. It's his problem, too, and his way of dealing is to focus, apparently, on how I'm dealing. But as usual, it'll be me in the hot seat, me on the table tolerating yet another invasive procedure, me with the restrictions on my activities until the pregnancy test ten days hence while Gary gets to go back to work like a normal person. It'll take all my resolve not to run out to Walgreens for a home pregnancy test, and when I read the result, I'll want to run back out for another to verify the findings.

The nice, older nurse has warned me not to succumb to this common craving. "There are too many false positives, and false negatives, before the full eleven days are up. You wouldn't want to get excited or disappointed for nothing. Trust me, waiting until we can perform the most accurate test is the biggest favor you'll do yourself in the next week and a half. That, and not doing anything that might cause you to blame yourself if the test is negative."

So I'll pass the time sublimating all my urges to drink coffee and beer, to eat certain types of cheese, to exercise, to sleep on my stomach (a personal bit of voodoo), all of these actions in case I'm pregnant, and then, when I'm not, I'll feel foolish for exhibiting false hope in the form of behavior modification and an imagined parental future.

"... in case you haven't noticed, there aren't any pictures of kids in Hamlin's office," Gary is saying. "In the hallway, yes, tacked up one on top of another, little girls with gigantic bows on their heads and baby boys dressed up like miniature Bears linebackers. But in his office? Not a one. Know why? Because he doesn't have any of his own, that's why. These women were talking about it on the elevator a couple of weeks ago. How he'd be the perfect dad, and what sort of major medical problem do you suppose he and his wife have that was beyond his incredible professional capacity to deal with. So if it's kids you want, which our present trip strongly suggests is the case, stick with unfashionable, sensible-car-driving-and-family-seeking me."

Dr. Hamlin loves me, or so he tells Gary as he stares up my crotch. I make him laugh, he says, to clarify he loves me not for my crotch. But I'm not feeling particularly funny this morning. Only nervous and worried and more than slightly mortified about how long it's been since my last bikini wax. I mean, who are all these people? All five of these men I've never seen?

They wear pistachio-colored scrubs, so I'll have to assume and hope that they're medical students or experienced IVF docs visiting from another country. There's no way they're bored dads on a break from the waiting room, I reassure myself, or Hamlin's poker buddies who won this experience when Hamlin added some interest to the pot at their weekly game. They have to be talented students or esteemed doctors who've seen this sort of thing hundreds of times before, barely even noticing I'm in the room, my exposed genitalia nothing more to them than any other domestic feature, blending in with the outlets and light switches and rolls of paper towels.

They're here to observe the great Kevin Hamlin, to note his outstanding medical technique and impressive bedside manner. It's astounding, really, the way he can carry on normal conversations and equipment checks mere inches from vaginas, unveiled and lit up like a Broadway show. I feel like the Taliban's enemy number one—both sets of hair on full and shameful display—and I yearn for somebody to hand me the world's heaviest, darkest, and most woolen burka.

Ask a question, I mentally beseech them. *Say something medical.* What I really want to do is announce, "Unless you care about what happens to me after this procedure, unless you can tell me my name, right now, first and last, unless you're hiding coffee cake somewhere in the drooping pockets of your baggy suits, unless one of you is packing a fertility phylactery, get the hell out of this room." But all I can muster is, "Looks like I'm double jointed."

The room is so wintry and the massive overhead spaceship of a lamp emits such a blitzkrieg of white light and red-hot heat that I lift my head to check for steam rising off of me. Dr. Hamlin has a gloved hand on my right thigh. "Just a couple more secs," he says, the warmth of his hand permeating the surgical glove. "The folks in the lab like to make sure, and make sure again, that the embryos they deliver are rightfully yours."

As we wait for the lab guys to carry in the loaded syringe, tipped up ceremonial phallus–style, Dr. Hamlin describes to the assembled group—medical practitioners and laypeople alike—his recent heli-skiing trip to the Italian and Swiss Alps. From my position, lying back on the table with my legs in the stirrups, his mouth looks like it's buried in my vagina. Each time he says the word *Alp*, I imagine he is lapping me up. *Alp. Alp. Alp.*

I've engaged my quads to keep my legs from splaying under the manual pressure. I'm shaking, too, because I'm uneasy and cold and working my leg muscles so hard and trying to make it look like I'm just kicking back, one relaxed lady enjoying a physician's yarn. I want to ask Dr. Hamlin to maybe release my leg, but I figure he's doing it for a reason—either to warm his hand, comfort me, or get his bearings. *If I place my hand at the exact center of the medial thigh portion, three and a half inches from the groin crease, and extend my thumb dorsally and draw a trajectory at a thirty-five-degree angle back toward the clitoris, I'll be able to position the catheter perfectly.*

There's a different nurse in here, too, an older one who is gentle and keen on explaining the procedures. I like her and decide that despite Gary's anxiously quiet presence in the room, she's my real partner for the moment. She's already told me that once they get going, it doesn't take long. She must realize that as hard as it is for women to hang out half nude in a room full of clothed people, it's even harder to do when you're in the dark.

A man calls from the next room—the embryo lab—that he has loaded our catheter with three nine-celled beauties. He walks in and asks me my name.

"Beth Kohl," I answer.

"Um. Uh-oh," he says. "Uh, Dr. Hamlin?"

"Liz. What name are you using here?" Dr. Hamlin asks. "The one you just gave doesn't sound right."

"Feinerman," Gary answers. "Elizabeth Feinerman. *F* as in Frank. *E-I-N-E-R-M-A-N.*"

"Phew," the lab guy whistles, handing the catheter over to Dr. Hamlin.

"Are we ready, George?" Dr. Hamlin asks. I'm relieved he's here. Good ol' George, with his Chicago Cubs scrub hat. "My wife gave me a box of those for our anniversary," he had explained when Gary complimented him. "She thought it was funny because *Cubs* and *scrubs* rhyme. I didn't have the heart to remind her I prefer the Sox. Not to mention the rhyming possibilities."

"Are we set, George?" Dr. Hamlin asks, pronouncing George's name the Spanish way.

"Ready, Hammy." George types in a few numbers and adjusts the ultrasound screen so Gary and I can see it, too. "We'll do a transabdominal ultrasound so Dr. H. can see where he's headed," he explains. "You'll notice a skinny bright line squirming through this here area." George places a cold plastic disk on my lower abdomen, and a series of shadows and brighter areas appear on the screen. He touches the monitor and traces a path with his finger. "Right here, as Dr. H. places the catheter. He'll let you know before he injects the embryos. Most people say it looks like a shooting star."

"Oh, great," I say. "I'd love to see that."

Gary stands behind me, his hand on my shoulder sweating through the thin, overlaundered cotton of my hospital gown. Dr. Hamlin busies himself, and we watch the image of the catheter creeping through me.

"Looks perfect," George tells Dr. Hamlin. "No. Maybe back it up a smidge."

"Okay?" Dr. Hamlin pulls his hand slightly. I feel the excess length of the catheter resting on my perineum and see the tip jiggle on the ultrasound screen.

"Yup. Perfect," George says.

"I'll release them now," Dr. Hamlin tells us. "Whoop. Did you catch that?"

I'm searching for a shooting star—a fixed one, even. I don't see a thing. "Yeah. I think I saw it." I'm afraid that maybe I lack the faith that allows those who succeed at this to do just that. Then I realize it's my first nanosecond of potential pregnancy, and I've ruined it with a lie.

On the eleventh day post-transfer, at two-thirty in the afternoon, the phone rings and I know it's Great Lakes calling with the results of the pregnancy test I'd taken that morning. Since the transfer, I've been living for this moment, imagining the conversation as I go about my days and lie down to sleep at night. I consider both ways it could go, one way starting with "Congratulations!" and the other with "I'm sorry." But mostly I consider the first eventuality, having every reason to believe that everything has gone perfectly and it'll work.

I pick up the phone, and it's Carol asking for me. I tell her yes, it's me. So? And in that split second between asking for the result and getting it, I know it is bad news. So I say, "You have bad news." And she says, "How can you tell?" And I say, "Okay. Thanks for calling." And she says, "Don't hang up. I need to give you some details." And I say, "I'm not really interested in the specifics of how unpregnant I am. Thanks anyhow," and hang up.

I call back later that afternoon. Carol is still there, and she takes my call.

"I know how tough it is to hear you're not pregnant, Elizabeth. Patients often forget the statistics and assume that every round will be a winning one. But you've only just begun, and if you'd like to try again in a couple of months, I can schedule it right now."

I tell her okay, that sounds fine. I also start crying, and she tells me I shouldn't cry, that things have looked pretty good for me all along but sometimes these things just don't work out, that as good as the science is and as accurate as the diagnostic tests are, embryos are simply unpredictable, and once they are inside the uterus, what goes on is anyone's guess.

How do I tell the story of the next few days, weeks, months? How do I account for our ability even to consider another round of infertility treatment after the disappointment and general sense of malaise? Oh, the visions I'd had, that swaddled, powdered baby so tantalizingly close, I could see his eyes flickering beneath his closed lids.

Worst was the lack of answers. Gary spoke of "inexact science" and spouted clichés about Mother Nature. My mom thought I hadn't prayed enough, while Gary's mother asked if I'd followed every last instruction: Had I accidentally forgotten some medicine or messed up the administration? As for Dr. Hamlin, whom I called before starting the next attempt, he reiterated that as good as my chances looked on paper, we couldn't forecast with any degree of certainty how I'd react to the meds until we'd actually tried them. He said he thought I needed higher doses of Gonal-F early on and that we'd played it too safe this time, forcing ourselves to play catch-up with immature eggs when my uterus had already peaked.

I took one month off—thirty-one days of rehashing all the ways I'd screwed up my chances, thinking to myself how alone I was in all this, hearing that this friend and that sister-in-law were expecting babies. I ran along the lakefront. I dug out this *Vogue Guide to Cocktails* book somebody had given us at our wedding shower and taught myself how to mix urbane drinks. Gimlets and martinis, things with Midori. I also avoided babies to the best of my ability, a difficult prospect when one lives en route to several of Chicagoland's favorite juvenile attractions.

Somewhat rejuvenated but a lot less enthusiastic, I returned to Highland Park for round two. The following month resembled round one, except I was sobered. When Gary voiced his concerns, I listened. We seriously discussed adopting a Chinese daughter. We agreed to learn the language and customs of her particular province and weave them into her American upbringing. I also found the Great Lakes Fertility staff infinitely more sympathetic and helpful this time. Perhaps I'd seemed too cocky the first round, oozing a naïve and insensitive eagerness to put off the staff. Or maybe I no longer cared about pleasing them, about what they thought of me. But how I was able to get through the logistics again, procuring the medicine, reconstituting the doses, and administering everything just so, I really can't say. I guess I just went on autopilot, kept my head down and my mouth shut, and went through the paces.

I had a good cycle, responding well to the drugs from the get-go. Upon aspiration, Dr. Hamlin was able to retrieve nineteen follicles, nine of which successfully fertilized. Debbie chose the three best blastocyst-stage embryos and froze the rest. After a day-five embryo transfer, I returned home to wait, and tried to lose myself in work and the lives of my friends and family. Eleven days later I returned to Great Lakes for an early morning blood test and received a call later that afternoon. I was pregnant.

Vernix Caseosa

By the end of March Chicago starts to thaw. I go out to our front stoop and inspect the yard, which appears intact if a bit thirsty. Only the crabapple tree hasn't survived; its exposed branches are like a prisoner caught, frozen, ashamed of his surrender. By now there should be some buds, a small leaf or two. Instead I discover an abandoned nest and a blue plastic bag trapped higher than I can reach.

Our neighbor, Mrs. DuBrul, cracks her front door for the first time in months, tearing a spiderweb that's advanced since November. One edge detaches and sags, weighted by leaf fragments and insect parts. I last saw Mrs. DuBrul in early January, shoveling her backyard. She labored over a path from the house to the garage, rebuking my offers to help.

"I may be old, but I'm not so decrepit I'd let a pregnant woman take over my chores." She coughed and scraped her chipped brown shovel against a thick layer of ice. Now she wears the marks of winter; her blue eyes are watery and red-rimmed, her skin is as flaky as baked phyllo.

I've had that baby, and at nine weeks she is sturdy enough to leave the house. In the hospital, the last week of January, a blizzard whorled outside the eleventh-floor window as I fought to conjure the infant Dr. Golden, my ob/gyn, had pulled from me and whisked, like stolen goods, onto my bare stomach. She smelled like rust, her skin looked like molten shellac, her fingers and toes were the color of a bruise. My neck ached as I strained to whisper, "Hello, I'm your mommy. All this time it's my voice you've been hearing," into her vernix-plugged ear.

This baby—induced two weeks early because the placenta was clogged, "like a dirty air filter," Golden had explained—gazed up in the direction of my face, stunned and rock still, while I issued telepathic commands. *Blink twice if you read me. Sigh once and curl your toes if I'm coming through.* The only movement came from Gary, who squeezed my shoulder and repeated, "Good job, hon. Way to go, hon. Hon, you did great."

Dr. Golden pushed down on my abdomen, warning that I'd feel a "whole lot of pressure. I'm delivering the afterbirth now," she reported. "I need to make sure the placenta is intact. You guys should pay attention to this part. It's something most people are too distracted to watch, and I'm assuming that, after all you've been through, you'll be interested in every last bit of the birthing process." She pressed her palms into me as if deflating a lifeboat. I felt my stomach collapse and heard a rush of liquid hit the tiled floor. "Yep. All here," she said, holding it up.

"Oy, God," Gary said. "Lovely."

A resident dropped iodine into the baby's eyes and asked what we'd decided to call her. The purple-black liquid dripped down her cheeks, marking her like Tammy Faye Bakker. We said we didn't know.

Despite the cumulative half-bottle of wine I had drunk in tiny glasses throughout my third trimester, the steaming baths I had sneaked, and all my fears about tinkering with Mother Nature, she appeared normal, for a newborn. Squish and swelling and molded head aside, she seemed not to be physically disfigured in any clinical way. I focused on her heart pounding against my belly, like a fingertip tapping a staccato beat from the inside.

A nurse wedged a latex-gloved hand between the baby and me, saying she needed to "borrow her," it would only be a minute or so. "What's your name?" she asked of the baby whose belly, I could now see, was coated with something off-white and swirly, like schmaltz. The nurse held her at arm's length, then placed her on the Ohio table. "What kind of name can there be for such a slimy girl?"

Of course there were possibilities. For the last three months Gary and I had discussed little else. And for the past two years I'd been keeping a mental tab, adding promising ones as I encountered them (Edie, Dahlia, Charlie) and taking others off the list as various celebs settled on them (Chloe, Aidan, Ava). I'd transcribed sixteen possible combinations, based on selections from *The New American Dictionary of Baby Names*, and organized them into columns according to whether we had a boy or girl, a blond, brunette, redhead, or bald baby, a baby-looking baby or more of an old person–looking baby. And now that we had met our daughter, now that she had rested on me and we had heard her yowl and seen the inside of her mouth, her gums unmarked as sea glass, none of the appellations fit. Names are for the civilized, the domesticated, the regulated. This infant was none of those. Of any being ever born, of all the tectonic plates crashing up into mountains, of all the Sistine Chapels and Easter Islands, *she* was inconceivable.

I peeled my wet gown from my skin, the thin cotton soaked like butcher paper, as the nurse talked to the baby across the room.

"We can't measure your color," she said, "what with all this cheese." She put down the pencil she'd been using to plot the baby's Apgar score.

"What 'cheese'?" Gary said, worried. "What do you mean, 'cheese'?"

"She's a couple weeks early, right?" the nurse asked. Cupping my silent infant's knit-capped head in one hand, she scooped some goo from the baby's baggy thigh. "This scummy stuff's *vernix caseosa*." She used her thumb to turn lubricated circles on her fingertips. "It waterproofs an unborn baby's skin. Once baby hits dry land, it's obsolete." She buffed her with a towel like a shoeshine man working a chamois.

"Hon. The nurse is sanding the baby. I don't like it."

Don't hurt her, I commanded silently. *Don't you dare hurt her.*

During our two postnatal days in the hospital, family and close friends streamed steadily through the electronic doors of the maternity ward and into my room, bringing velour outfits for the baby, sushi for me. Unlikely people showed up, too. The next-door neighbors I occasionally called hello to over the back fence, at the hospital for flu shots so why not stop up, say hello, meet the new neighbor. An art school classmate I liked but hardly knew who brought a stuffed animal and balloon arrangement so blimplike we couldn't stop it from traveling, willy-nilly, around the room and stopping up the doorway. Gary managed to shepherd them all out by warning that the longer they hung around, the worse off they'd be, snow-wise.

Alone, I wondered whether being born during a blizzard, like marrying in the rain or getting shat on by a bird, was good luck. A nurse rapped on my half-closed door, made her way over to my bed, and fastened a blood pressure cuff around my upper arm.

"They say Eskimos unwrap their newborns," she told me,

looking out the window and pumping the cuff way too tight, "and hold them, naked, in the cold air for a few minutes every day for the first three weeks."

"Why's that?" I asked.

She turned a dial and let the air out before loudly ripping the cuff from my arm. "You know, I can't really say. Maybe they think it'll ward off evil spirits. Either that or to promote circulation."

"Nigerian fishermen plunge their newborn babies into the river and let them flounder kind of until the last moment." I had heard this from a cabdriver. "You know, until the baby stops waving its arms and legs and rolls over, facedown, in the water."

"No kidding," she said. "But really, that's not the same thing I'm talking about. That's not superstitious or healthy. That's just reckless."

On our front stoop I sit holding the two-month-old child I've cocooned inside a down snowsuit that's too big and, over that, a thick wool blanket. The baby sleeps in my arms. Her head, pulled long by the slow labor, rounded out after a day or two. Her lips are full, like mine, and her eyes are feline and over-sized, like her father's. Her only blemish is her ears, which are pinched at the top, the tubular ridge along the upper edge a blot on the rest of her.

One block west, across the street, is a hospital for children. Children's Memorial Hospital. What a preposterous combina-tion, these words. As lunatic a coupling as ever there was, like *necrophilia* or *rice cake*.

Just outside our front gate women push children in wheel-chairs down the sidewalk. Some of them are nurses. I can tell by their gummy white clogs and light green cotton pants. The others must be moms, propelling massive, complicated chairs toward the lake, maneuvering to avoid ice patches and cracks in the cement. Many of the children's heads are propped up by metal tongs, like collectible dolls. Several look around at the houses in this strange neighborhood they've been living in. A few talk to the women who push them, their high-pitched voices cutting through the air as they babble of McDonald's and soccer, fooling me into thinking for a moment that they're like any of the children I see on our street, the one that leads to the zoo, the nature museum, and the beach.

Foil balloons knotted to the backs of the chairs snap in the wind. One of them bangs into a woman's shoulder with a hollow ting as she hits a crevice in front of Mrs. DuBrul's house.

"Goddamn it all," the lady says, walking around to the front of the chair. "You okay, Pickle Bug?"

"I'm fine, Ma," says a boy. He's wearing flannel pants and a Green Bay Packers jacket that's too small. Maybe it fit the last time he wore it. His ma wears a similar jacket. These two are a team. They should have their own name and mascot. The Braves. The Grayskins. The Oakland Y's.

"You sure?" she asks.

"I said I'm fine."

I think I might be staring. They see me and follow my glance as I look away. I strain not to look down at my baby. I try to seem casual, a new mother taking advantage of the break in the weather, minding her own business.

Pickle Bug's ma manages to extricate the stuck tire by popping a wheelie. They continue down the street, small mounds of snow flanking their way. The boy's head is swollen like a lopsided water balloon. He probably can't so much as walk around the block on his own. He can't go outside, maybe anywhere, without tubes to externally perform the functions that the rest of us perform on the inside, by ourselves. And his mother asks if he's fine. What does he know from fine?

Fine is what I want my baby to be. *Fine* is what I want IVF to be in the long run. *Fine* is what I want Sophia to say when I explain to her how we went about having her. *Fine*—such a blasé response, the word of the insincere and the casual, of acceptance and understanding, just tell me everything will be fine and I'll be okay.

I sneak into Sophia's room while she sleeps, see her arms stretched overhead like field-goal posts, and hold my breath. She's already outgrown the tiny things of hers I've been embarrassed to pronounce—footies and onesies and passies—even though it's been only nine weeks since I sterilized and laundered and folded them just so in the changing table. The amphibian curl of her legs, last vestige of her in utero pose, unfurls with each passing day. They'll straighten and she'll use them, walk and run and kneel on them, until they're crooked again. But I won't be around for that.

The thought interrupting my sleep is the same one that allows this kid, Pickle Bug, to wake up in the morning, swallow food, and quiet his ma. This—my house, Chicago's potholed streets, the wheels on his chair, my child's seventh week, Mrs. DuBrul—all of this is only temporary.

And these women. What's wrong with these women? How merciless to flaunt this beautiful day! How dare they let these children lay eyes on the rest of us, those who've somehow survived to adulthood, who get to drive a car, dig up dead trees, have kids of our own! I can only guess they must hope the air will do the kids some good. Ward off evil spirits. Promote circulation.

I hear a voice. "Ma'am," it says. "Ma'am." I look up. A nurse is at the front gate. "May we see the baby? Josie loves babies."

She stands beside a contraption, half-chair, half-gurney, with a girl laid out on it, her bald head immobilized in a fleece-wrapped metal ring, her eyes wrenched to the side. She could be six. Or maybe she's twelve. Her nose runs, and a thread of drool traces a shivery line between her mouth and an armrest, but the nurse doesn't notice, focused as she is on my daughter. The last thing I want is to allow my child contact with whatever is wrong with that girl, but I don't say no. How can I say no?

Slowly I get up. I unwrap Sophia's blanket, pull it taut, and tuck it, tight as a tourniquet, around every inch not needed for breathing. I step down the stairs and cross the front walk until I'm standing just on our side of the gate. I adjust Sophia, who feels as heavy as an encyclopedia, so that her head rests in the crook of my arm. Josie lifts both hands into the air, her fingers opening and closing like a toddler's wave. An IV tube swings, arcing between one thin, translucent arm and a metal rod that juts from the back of her conveyance. I open the gate, bend down, offer Sophia toward her, and whisper "Let's not wake the baby" into her perfect ear.

Sophia proved herself a good baby, eating when presented food, cooing when held or mugged at, sleeping when placed in her crib. There was no colic, not one sleepless night. I nursed her without pain or incident, believing in the La Leche League message, if not its guerrilla tactics. I nursed her in bathrooms and clothes-store changing rooms, I nursed her at home until we'd both doze off, the two of us in her room at odd hours, rocking in an overstuffed chair while tree branches knicked the window.

But I worried things were going too smoothly. Not only had I breezed through my pregnancy, eating untold numbers of burgers, platters of cheesy eggs, and dollops of ranch dressing yet mustering only a ten-pound weight gain (expelling six pounds, eleven ounces with the birth of Sophia), I loved being pregnant. I felt energized by and connected to my gestating child. My transition to motherhood had been just as easy. In no way did I feel changed in any essential way. Certainly I felt a new and overpowering sense of responsibility, an intense bond and thrilling love. But the person who had decided in the first place to become a mother seemed to have survived the whole process. From the protracted attempts to the actual conception through the nine months and the labor and delivery, I still felt like me.

Indeed, having a baby produced in me a deep satisfaction and sense of relief: not only that I could have a baby but that I loved being her mother. I'd worried I wouldn't feel that way. I worried that having a baby after struggling so much for it would be anticlimactic. I worried that overwhelming guilt—for bringing a child into this world, for exposing her to potential IVF-related health risks, for creating a child who might blame herself if I end up succumbing to an IVF-implicated ovarian or uterine cancer—would get in the way of happiness. But I was overjoyed with my daughter; her every crevice and hollow exactly as it should be, her velveteen head and sweet-sour smell so prototypically baby.

"Why do you pore over her like that?" Gary asked me one night, after I'd bathed Sophia in the kitchen sink, then lotioned and powdered her on the countertop, the pajamas in a small pile next to her makeshift changing table as I held up her arms and legs and pressed my ear to her back to listen to the internal noises. "Looking for something specific?"

"I'm just checking," I said. "I want to know as much about her as I can. I think it's normal for a new mother."

Truth was, as much as I enjoyed the hunt, I thought if I looked hard enough I might discover the place where IVF was etched on her. Was it the flattened ears? Would we get off that easily?

I'd take Sophia to the pediatrician for baby-wellness checks, where she consistently maintained her percentiles, fortieth for weight, sixty-fifth for length, fiftieth for head circumference. The office was on the third floor of a building next to the El, the exam rooms lined up in a row overlooking the tracks. Parents would hear the train coming and say, "Here comes the choo choo. Look at the pretty choo choo," to their crying or sullen or nervous kids. We'd go to the windows, holding our babies and toddlers in our arms, waving and watching as passengers mutually distracted by us whizzed noisily by.

A nurse would come in, carrying Sophia's file. She'd ask me to strip Sophia down to her diaper, and she'd weigh her on a plastic, scooped-out scale like at the deli counter. She'd stretch Sophia's legs on the paper-covered exam table, hold down the crown of her head, and make pencil marks at the top and bottom. She'd wrap a tape measure around Sophia's head and jot down the findings. She'd interpret the results, tracing the measurements to somewhere smack dab in the chart's middle.

Relieved to have an easily quantifiable child, still I'd think about Darwin and subtle human differences and wacko theories such as Jimmy the Greek's proposition about slave-breeding techniques impacting modern-day athletics, Nazis and eugenics and studies plotting the correlation between head circumference and mental ability. Were IVF babies a new category of physically distinct beings, I wondered, with a mark, like the thumbprint of a potter, on their scientifically enabled form? Would they excel at certain activities, at glassblowing or statistics or life drawing, and falter at others, at earthy natural ones like organic farming or reproducing?

I dressed Sophia thoughtfully, avoiding anything vaguely scratchy or cutesy. I made sure I knew how to buckle her securely into car seats and strollers, how to collapse all of her various gear—the Pack-n-Play, the Combi City Savvy Select Stroller, the baby jogger, and the sun tent—to fit into the back of our new, more spacious car. I felt like a normal mom, forgetting a little with time how much I'd struggled to achieve motherhood. I looked like the other mothers, sensibly dressed, hair in a ponytail, a vaguely fashionable diaper bag slung over my shoulder.

We'd go to Wiggleworms, to Mommy and Me. I sang words from my childhood as Sophia, distracted by the other babies, ignored me. I'd row her arms and make bicycle circles with her legs. I'd kiss the top of her head over and over and put her on her tummy at regular intervals and to sleep on her back at night, just as the surgeon general recommended.

All in all, she wasn't a big smiler. I mentioned it to the pediatrician, Dr. Cane, who explained it wasn't a cause for concern. She's clearly attentive and interacts with her surroundings, even if not jollily. He admitted she seemed serious, adding that some of the most successful people aren't exactly giddy.

"Look at Ruth Bader Ginsburg and Alan Greenspan," he said. "Look at Ralph Nader."

"But her father and I are both laughers."

"Maybe she'll lighten up," Dr. Cane said. "Maybe not."

I told the doctor I admired his laid-back attitude but kept on wondering whether Sophia was really destined to be sullen or if IVF had impaired her joyfulness, if the ICSI needle had perforated the happiness gene on its way on in. Thankfully, by the time she turned one, she started breaking out into heartbreaking smiles, at squirrels and at the dog, at her dada and me, whom she called Beth, like a stepmother.

As Sophia grew, she revealed a fantastic imagination, a staggering memory, a quirky and charming personality. We considered ourselves the luckiest parents in the world, cosmically blessed and somehow excused from normal new-parent problems as a gift from the same universe that had made conception so difficult. We had a good run, two whole years, in fact, without so much as a sniffle. But then one day, just as I was walking in from having dropped Sophia off, I received a phone call from St. Chrysostom's, Sophia's preschool. Before answering, I prayed it would be an administrator, somebody telling me our hefty tuition check had bounced or that Sophia's backpack, the miniature fuchsia one to which I hot-glued felt ricrac and a Liberty-print name tag, had gone missing, anything but news that there was something wrong with our problem-free daughter.

"Mrs. Feinerman?" Sophia's teacher, Mrs. Kerry, said. "It's Joyce Kerry. I don't mean to alarm you, but I believe Sophia has had a seizure. The children were in the gym, and I happened to glance up just as Sophia walked toward me, and I could swear, she was seizing. You know, dead in her tracks, eyes vibrating back and forth in her head, totally not in control of what was happening and unresponsive when I called her name. I think you should come and get her and head right to the emergency room."

Pulling out into traffic, I assured Sophia that everything was all right, we just needed to go check something at the hospital. I cranked the children's music CD on heavy rotation in our car and called Gary.

"It's that fucking man-made brain," I said, crying all of a sudden and hoping Sophia was listening to the Grand Old Duke of York. "Her whole body, it's like a house of cards just waiting to blow over."

"Her brain is not man-made," Gary said. "She's a regular person, just like anybody else. As long as she spent the requisite amount of time gestating, she's perfectly healthy. That is, unless she has epilepsy, which would be terrible but not the end of the world. We'll deal with what life brings, right?"

The brain scans and sleep deprivation studies showed no sign of epilepsy. No other problems, either. Perhaps the seizures had been febrile, the pediatric neurologist reasoned, even though I'd told them, the pediatricians, over and over that she'd had no fever that day. Perhaps they were anomalous, an innocent and isolated electrical misfiring, something that kids sometimes experience and that, in most cases, never recurs. She hadn't suffered a stroke and absolutely, positively didn't have epilepsy. I was comforted, too, that experts had had the opportunity to pore over pictures of her brain and, rather than flinching or flagging anything, tossed the X-rays aside like any other case that no longer holds interest.

More troubling were the emergency surgeries needed to remove a couple of urachal cysts, embryonic structures connecting the fetal bladder to what eventually becomes the umbilical cord. In Sophia's case, the urachus never filled, remaining open and prone to infection. Sophia's first cyst was attached to the underside of her navel, hovering just beneath the surface of her skin like a man-o'-war. I noticed her belly button protruding and assumed it was a hernia, a common problem in my family and ultimately no big deal. I took her to see Dr. Cane, who pressed on it with his thumb to try to reduce it. As it popped back out, he said it looked suspiciously unhernialike, that its size, shape, and consistency were more typical of a cyst. He ordered an abdominal ultrasound at Children's Memorial, called a surgeon he particularly liked, and told us to head right over, they'd be expecting us.

The ultrasound turned up the anticipated cyst, and we met that afternoon with a pediatric surgeon named Dr. Jennings, who recommended surgery since it looked to be infected. She operated the next day, removing it and noting post-op that it had been superficial and easily accessible, showing us on a sleeping Sophia's belly the tiny incision she had had to make. "The scar will be negligible," she assured us. Did we look like we cared about scars? "The skin on her navel might pucker a bit on the side I cut, but if you have to have a scar, that's a pretty darn good spot."

"There goes her career as a stripper," Gary said. Dr. Jennings smiled.

"As long as I was in there," she continued, "I thought it'd be wise to scrape the surrounding tissue, just to assure we got it all. We'll have to watch for infection, but it really went fine. She did great."

"Thank you, Dr. Jennings," Gary and I said in unison. "Thank you so much," he repeated.

Then almost a year later we went to Disneyland. We left L.A., where we were staying with my brother David and his family, early in the morning and drove the forty-five miles southward, past the car dealerships and the palm trees, past the big-box stores with the giant inflated gorillas on their roofs. Sophia complained of a stomachache in the backseat.

"She's just hungry," Gary reasoned. "Once we get there and she gets a load of all that great junk food, she'll be fine."

We drove the rest of the way to Anaheim and parked in the Pinocchio lot, then boarded the tram into Disneyland proper and walked around the park. I kept a close eye on Sophia, gauging whether her stomach still bothered her and trying to see whether she was enjoying these Disney things I'd so loved as a kid.

"Come on," I said, trying to goad her into acting delighted, "this is fun. I loved all this stuff when I was your age. You know, I still have the necklace my mom bought me when I came here. The one with the beaded Native American princess? I don't think you realize how special this trip is for all of us, Sophia." I left her on the sidewalk with Gary as I shopped for the things I knew I would like if I was still three.

We'd saved It's a Small World for last, embarking on a boat and floating through a warehouse filled with mechanized children of the world singing the same song over and over. Their half-moon eyelids blinked with audible clicks, and the Tahitian girls danced in a circle, shaking their hips so fast the shells on their skirts never touched down. Sophia grabbed her stomach and held her breath as a fezzed kid in pointy shoes hovered overhead on a bent carpet.

"Gary," I said, "I think Sophia might really be sick."

I tried to figure out an escape route, a means of hastening the ride's end. But there was no outboard motor, no set of oars, no panic button. I held a listless Sophia in my lap as Dutch and African and Thai robot kids stomped their clogs and danced to drums and rode around on yaks. One last tour through Scandinavia, and the ride was over, our boat rear-ending the ones in front of it. Telling Gary I'd meet him at the restroom entrance, we climbed out, rushed through the gift shop (the only egress), retrieved our stroller from the stroller corral, and raced into the bathroom, choosing a handicapped stall to accommodate me, Sophia, the stroller, and our assorted Disney swag—Finding Nemo plush toys, two plasticky nightgowns with substantial pointy "jewels" sewn to their fronts, and a pair of light pink Mouseka-ears, which a smiling Disney employee had personalized for Sophia while I waited.

On the way back to L.A. I sat in back with Sophia, holding her hand and urging Gary to drive faster, this as he struggled not to dent his father-in-law's fender, this as I silently prayed not only that my daughter would be all right but that she'd not puke in the back of Gary's father-in-law's car.

My brother called to say he'd gotten us in with his pediatrician, who'd made it clear he normally didn't see nonpatients but liked my brother's adorable son so well he'd make this one exception. The doctor couldn't pinpoint the problem but recommended we eliminate wheat and dairy from Sophia's diet and suggested that her fever could be her body's way of fighting off infection. "Nature's furnace functioning on cue," he said. We booked a flight back to Chicago and left early the next morning, heading directly from the airport to the hospital.

Not wanting to mess around after our last experience, Dr. Cane ordered another abdominal ultrasound, which revealed a dramatically larger cyst attached along its length to Sophia's bladder. Dr. Jennings met us that afternoon in an exam room, a gigantic envelope presumably containing the new ultrasound images in hand. She shook Sophia's hand, said hello to me and Gary, nice to see you again, sorry about the circumstances, and headed over to a radiology viewbox mounted on the wall.

Sophia had surgery later that day, this time requiring a hip-to-hip incision, while Gary and I sweated it out in a family waiting room. A phone on the wall would ring as different children emerged from surgery. There was no stated protocol for answering it, no posted flyer in a festive font with stock graphics like in other parts of the hospital, so we family members took turns, depending on who was closest or awake or not too distraught. After a couple of hours the phone rang and a Polish man answered and called out, "Feinerman," and I said, "That's us," and hurried to the phone. "Your daughter's out of surgery. Room three," somebody said.

Dr. Jennings was waiting in a small anteroom connected to an OR. Through glass windows I could see people arranging ribbed tubes and multicolored cords and blinking machines around an impossibly small, knocked-out, and inanimate-looking Sophia. The doctor explained the procedure and what it had yielded. She had needed to make a rather large incision, a truly stripper-career-compromising one, and had removed the entire, clearly infected cyst and some surrounding tissue, but in no way had she impacted Sophia's bladder. She apologized for missing the second cyst the first go-round, and we told her we didn't blame her. She continued that, upon reflection, she should have followed up the first operation with a more thorough exam. "Maybe this cyst would have been enlarged, maybe not," she said, "but I bet I could have caught it."

Stop beating yourself up, doc, I wanted to say. *It's not your fault. You're not dealing with a normal physique here. Sophia is an IVF baby, so of course there are going to be physical anomalies.* I didn't say anything, not even to Gary when we were sitting in Sophia's hospital room the next day and he mentioned that he thought the doctor might have been negligent. But I couldn't dismiss the fact that our daughter had had a rare problem in an anatomical structure so closely connected to embryonic life and that her body had thrown for a loop this most experienced of pediatric surgeons.

IVF babies have been born in this country since 1981, but questions remain about what health impact the reproductive technology might have on them, from infancy on through to adulthood. Studies yield conflicting results. Dr. Howard Jones, the man who enabled the first American IVF baby's conception, had prepared two alternate statements to read the day she was born. The first was to be read in case of disfigurement or any other indication that she wasn't completely normal. The other was in case she appeared to be okay. Luckily, he got to read the latter. But that's not to say problems can't be hidden or dormant, only that little Elizabeth Carr looked perfectly Martian, just like any normal newborn.

Of the three hundred or so published reports involving children conceived using ART, some show IVF-enabled children to be no different, health-wise, from their naturally derived peers, while others have raised serious concerns. One Australian study found that babies conceived through IVF or ICSI (check, check) were more than twice as likely as naturally conceived infants to have a major birth defect (9 versus 3 percent), particularly heart problems and urinary- and genital-tract issues.

In 2002 The New England Journal of Medicine published a study that found IVF children more than twice as likely as naturally conceived children to have been diagnosed with a major birth defect by age one. They were also more likely to require delivery by C-section, be born preterm, and have a low birth-weight. Subsequent studies not only confirmed these findings but added some terrible things to the list, including a greater propensity for certain cancers such as retinoblastoma (a childhood cancer arising from immature retinal cells in one or both eyes that can strike from the time a baby is in the womb up to five years of age) and for urogenital problems.

Researchers from Washington University and Johns Hopkins studied children who had Beckwith-Wiedemann syndrome (BWS), an overgrowth disorder that causes enlarged organs, abdominal wall defects, gigantism, and an increased risk for developing cancerous tumors. They found a disproportionate number of IVF children among their sample. BWS is thought to be caused by an alteration in a child's genes, and even though it is often inherited, other cases are classified as new mutations.

Some doctors think BWS may be caused by ICSI. Injecting a sperm directly into an egg for fertilization may interfere with imprinting, the switching on and off of genes in the earliest days of embryonic development. Certainly introducing the tip of a sperm-carrying pipette into an egg has to leave some mark, however infinitesimal. I often wished we could have accomplished this step otherwise, using an all-natural substance (how about semen?) or subcontracting to a magician. The Amazing Art would enter the operating room, his magician's cape, hat, and scarf fashioned out of that light blue polyester that most doctor's exam coats are made of. He'd take the egg dish in one gloved hand and the dish of sperm in the other. *Sim sala bim*, he'd say, tipping the sperm dish to reveal it was now empty. The nurse would aim the OR lights at his other hand, illuminating the shadows of thrashing-tailed sperm swimming inside the eggs. A couple of balloon shapes—a sperm for the gentlemen, fallopian tubes for the ladies, or vice versa—and he'd be out of there.

In fact, a study out of Johns Hopkins Children's Center in 2003 reported that a group of rare urological defects, including bladder development outside the body, could be more common in IVF children. The Johns Hopkins research looked at seventy-eight children with cloacal-bladder exstrophy-epispadias complex, a condition in which the bladder is exposed, inside out, and protrudes through the abdominal wall, who'd received treatment at Johns Hopkins from 1998 to 2001. The research found that IVF children have a seven times higher incidence of this birth defect than children in the general population. And while Sophia certainly hadn't had that complex, she'd had a bladder-related problem that hinted, at least to the mother who is still surprised each time she sees her daughter's deeply scarred belly, at the full-blown disease.

"What we are seeing now is simply an association between this group of birth defects and IVF births," said the Hopkins study's senior author, John P. Gearhart, director of the division of pediatric urology at the Children's Center. "Further research is needed to verify those findings and understand this association. These defects are extremely rare, and our preliminary findings should not alone discourage couples from undergoing IVF."

A CDC study shows that full-term singletons conceived through ART, no matter the specific procedure, were more than twice as likely as infants in the general population to be born underweight (6.5 percent versus 2.5 percent). Other studies linked ICSI with Angelman syndrome, a condition that can cause developmental problems and speech impairment. The ASRM, at its 2004 conference, conducted a workshop exploring whether IVF babies are at greater risk for developing certain chromosomal and genetic abnormalities and, if so, whether doctors have a professional, moral, or ethical duty to warn their patients.

The researchers wonder whether it's the disease (infertility) or its treatments (ART) that cause the observed defects. That is, do infertile couples who undergo ART have characteristics, the defective eggs and sperm a symptom of a larger problem or a significant defect in and of themselves, that place them at greater risk of having children with abnormalities? Some believe that the drugs and the procedures cause the damage—the medications used to stimulate the ovaries or maintain the pregnancy, to freeze and thaw embryos, or the insertion of a needle into the egg during ICSI. Dr. Arnold Strauss, chief of pediatrics at Vanderbilt University Medical Center in Nashville and a member of a U.S. panel analyzing the data, explained the theoretical risk posed by ART procedures: "The speculation would be that you're dealing with cells that are put into conditions that they would never normally see."

Experts commenting on the studies emphasize that the observed abnormalities are uncommon to begin with and remain so even if the risk is magnified several times. Many of the problems also stem from common multiplicity issues, complications associated with multiple births in general rather than specifically with ART. As Dr. Strauss said, "Common sense would say that a lot of people have been through this and most of their children are doing well. It's really a question of subtlety and small differences."

Plenty of other studies conclude that IVF babies have no increased threat of health complications, no greater risk of birth defects or developmental disorders, of ADD or autism, debunking the idea that natural fertilization is the one true path to ideal health and maximized human capacity. Judging from my kids—Sophia, and the two sisters, Anna and Lily, who followed—the way this one can color for hours at a time, how that one can do chin-ups like a Navy SEAL, I'd have to proclaim them perfectly typical. They're developing normally, age-appropriately, and suffer as many sniffles and tumbles and disappointments and nightmares as the kid-population at large. They love imaginative play and ice cream, and hate asparagus and bedtime, like any kid. So like any parent, birth or adoptive, foster or step, I'll do my best to protect them from preventable harm and help them navigate life's unavoidable conflicts— and I'll keep my fingers way crossed.

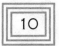

10

Fertility Karma

On August 18, 1992, Courtney Love gave birth to Frances Bean Cobain. In November of the prior year, one presumes that Ms. Love and her then-boyfriend, rocker Kurt Cobain, in a rush of chemical euphoria, conceived their baby. Whether backstage after a Nirvana concert, warming up for a Hole act, or rather more quotidian—the missionary position atop a Posturepedic mattress—they had sex, she conceived. A *Vanity Fair* article that year reported that Love used heroin while pregnant. She claimed that she stopped after realizing she was pregnant.

In the spring of 2001, a few months shy of an apparently healthy Frances Bean's eighth birthday, and two months after I'd once again started up my own drug-heavy regimen, albeit a prescribed and legitimately acquired one, Dr. Kevin Hamlin launched, for the fourth time, three blastocyst-stage embryos into my uterus. As I dressed post-transfer, I pictured the cellular clusters floating slowly, perhaps taking tentative hold.

Finally, after the months of constant appointments and shots and ultrasounds and blood draws, after the years of medical diagnoses, the aborted and failed cycles, and the successful cycle that resulted in beautiful Sophia, I once more had fertilized embryos inside my body, just like anybody else, just like Courtney Love.

From my unsuccessful previous attempts and my awareness of IVF statistics, I knew better than to consider the embryos cemented in. With a less than 50 percent success rate even for women under thirty-five who use their own fresh eggs, I could only presume the embryos were unstable and easily perturbed. But look at the odds that Ms. Love's conception and eventual fetus had surmounted. Not only had Love conceived, she'd actually ingested heroin, and presumably while doing other not-so-good-for-her things. It wasn't that she'd heaved grocery bags, consumed too many ounces of mercurous tuna fish, admitted to enjoying Caesar dressing, sushi, carpaccio, feta cheese, cunnilingus, or other pregnancy no-nos. She'd done crank, hazel, Mexican brown. Whatever you called it, 'twas not folic acid.

There is a common refrain heard within the fertility trenches, a general riff on one's cursed luck even while undeserving wretches drown in fertility bounty. Sitting in a waiting room and tuning in to the conversations, or fielding a fellow patient's commentary, one is apt to hear about the inequity, the shocking unfairness of it all.

"James and I met during our Rhodes scholarships while completing graduate work in fetal wellness," the complaints essentially go. "We bonded over our mutual respect for the gestating human. After spending a decade working with pregnant mothers in rural Africa, we came back to the States, established our pediatric practice, and moved into a one hundred percent lead-free home selected in large part for its proximity to the finest public-school district in the nation. For the past two years, before going to work to take care of other peoples' babies, I've been coming to Great Lakes for early-morning blood draws and ultrasounds. I'm on my fifth round of IVF, this while welfare mothers and crack whores and teenagers, *teen-agers*, who'd do anything *not* to be pregnant again, just can't seem to prevent their well-functioning reproductive bodies from functioning well. Where's the justice? If there's a God, and all those hours I've spent kneeling in church make me want to believe there is, why is He testing our faith? If there's a God, why doesn't He want us to have a baby, preferring welfare mothers and crack whores and *teenagers* to a couple of sensibly housed and gainfully employed pediatricians?"

To be fair, Love and Cobain were in their late twenties when they had their baby, pulling down a substantial income, and more into junk than crack, really. But they'd had the benefit of innocent reproductive sex, they'd enjoyed recklessness and, perhaps, something hot, hot, hot, this as I considered how many people had witnessed my own conception attempts, and none of them roadies. Unlike me, all it took for Courtney and Kurt was an ounce or two of heroin and some old-fashioned, if somewhat grungy, sex.

After the procedure, Gary holds my forearm as I shuffle back to our curtained room. I don't really need his help, but I like having that extra bit of support as the clock starts ticking on the waiting period until I am to return for a pregnancy test. I dread the moment of sitting down, it being the first of many compromises I will expose my heretofore clinically managed embryos to. Having vowed to take more control over this crucial portion of the cycle, I sheath the patient chair with a spare hospital gown and slowly, deliberately lower myself to a variation on sitting.

Handing over the pile of clothes I'd shakily removed earlier that morning, Gary looks on in a silent admonition, or so I take it, not to bungle things. I push my arms through the three-quarter-length sleeves of my T-shirt. How asinine this item now seems, how silly the heavy gray sweatpants, an ideal outfit for a Little Leaguer but surely inappropriate for somebody harboring three tiny miracles. What I need is a suit of armor or something soft and quilted and puffy. What I need is baby bunting. Better yet, this momentous occasion calls for ceremonial vestment—a kimono, or my wedding dress. What about that good-luck charm bracelet my mom gave me before I left for college? The four-leaf clover and horseshoe charms, the disembodied hand with its crossed fingers and the cloisonné carp pinging as I moseyed around campus, wrote papers, and threw back yards of beer? Hey, where's Gary's yarmulke? Why hadn't I thought to bring a piece of my largely unworn bridal lingerie at the very least, a private token buried beneath the thoughtless array of deeply discounted cotton wear from a final clearance rack at the Gap?

I need to tie my shoelaces, but I fear bending over will generate more uterine stress than raising my foot and resting it on the chair's edge. But I can't ask Gary to perform such a menial task, not after he's just witnessed Hamlin's extraordinary works. So I lift my feet slowly, ever so slowly, and tie my shoes. I think about how much I loved being pregnant before. How entertaining it was to try to figure out if I was carrying a boy or girl without ever succumbing to technology for a definitive answer. My tastes changed as well, and I look fondly back on my first trimester as a time of rekindling my long-extinguished love affair with beef. During that time I enjoyed swimming, the exhilarating buoyancy on my increasingly earthbound body. I bought books on pregnancy that explained the evolution of the maternal and fetal bodies throughout the forty weeks and studied what the gestating baby looked like on any particular day. Day thirty-six? Two millimeters long, with burgeoning ears and rounded eyes like pushpins. Day hundred and one? Three and a half inches long. With a neck! And fingerprints!

I had unbelievable surges of energy, organizing the house and filing receipts, cleaning closets and scrubbing baseboards. I fit an extra workshop into my school schedule and chiseled out extra gym time, taking spinning classes and toning my arms and legs even as my belly swelled. Women, older ladies on treadmills, would interrupt their own workouts to tell me how great I looked, the picture of maternal health. As long as I wore a heart rate monitor and kept my body temperature and heart rate at safe levels, Dr. Golden, who I'd bump into at the gym, said moderate exercise was beneficial.

So I know from experience that I can get through a pregnancy with flying colors, and a somewhat protracted and typically painful delivery even, with a healthfully crying baby to show for it. But now, when the all-too-delicate embryos have been introduced and require a perfectly stable environment in which to take hold and continue to develop, this is the hard part. I'll need to provide two weeks of calm, a dozen doses of progesterone served up in suppository form, trips to Great Lakes for continued monitoring, and some nontechnological positive thinking, an indispensable complement to the science.

Last night, I taped Great Lakes' post-transfer instructions to our kitchen cabinet. If I follow them exactly—lay down for a few hours of strict bed rest upon returning post-transfer, followed by two more days of moderated bed rest (lying on the couch is okay, but climbing stairs more than once a day or doing other excessive domestic activity is not), don't swim or take a bath or douche or use tampons or drive for a couple of days or strain to lift heavy objects or jog or do aerobics or play tennis or have intercourse or an orgasm—until a fetal heartbeat appears on the ultrasound (or until a pregnancy test is negative), everything will be fine. Not that I ever would want to have sex or an orgasm, play tennis, or engage in any other brisk leisure activity ever again if the pregnancy test is negative.

At some point Carol reassures me that while implanted embryos are somewhat fragile, masses of pregnant people in the general, non-ART population go about their normal business each and every day. They booze it up and enjoy hydrogenated oils, they go to work and ski, lift weights and heavy children, and end up with healthy pregnancies and babies in the pink. Still, I'm afraid I'll somehow mess up Hamlin's great and careful work with my clumsiness, driving to the grocery store out of habit and mindlessly loading up the shopping cart with cases of water and sacks of dog food. Only after returning from this errand would I spot the posted sheet, the highlighted lines about not driving, not lifting heavy items, blurring through my tears.

I keep in mind the Jell-O mold image: the embryos suspended somehow (how?) and not just free-floating, spastically bouncing all over the place or slamming into one another. I think of how nature and evolution have so perfectly equipped the human body for reproductive success. Ah, and scientific genius, advanced medicine—these magnificent buttresses for bodies requiring reinforcement. But, if out-of-control types, body and drug abusers, if dinosaur-bone-hauling cavewomen and occasionally tumbling trapeze artists manage to get pregnant, why couldn't relatively clean-living, feet-on-the-ground, and medically enhanced I? If I not only laze calmly around the house but also boost the embryos with luteal-phase support in the form of estrogen tablets and progesterone suppositories those first crucial days, if I steer clear of stresses to the body, don't pick up Sophia, and refuse all Kamikaze shots, surely I'll be ahead of the game.

Then again, the very real potential for failure is why some doctors readily transfer upward of six embryos a pop. A 2005 study by the Yale School of Medicine published in *Fertility and Sterility* concluded that 85 percent of embryos transferred during IVF fail to become live births. Dr. Pasquale Patrizio, the professor in the ob/gyn department who led the research, concluded that better methods for predicting embryonic viability are needed, such as "pre-implantation genetic diagnosis and biochemical markers of embryo viability." He also hoped his study would move the reproductive technology field toward "perfecting methods of egg production."

Doctors have tried to develop an embryo-classification system to help predict pregnancy chances. But the work is imprecise and based largely on subjective measures, visible criteria like degree and patterns of fragmentation. As it stands, embryos are graded according to their appearance and rate of cell division. The best-quality embryos are called Grade A, like at the dairy, and must have between four and eight cells of equal size, clear cytoplasm, and few fragments (pieces of cytoplasm in the zona pellucida, the strong membrane that forms around an ovum as it develops and that remains in place until fertilization occurs, disappearing completely to permit implantation in the uterus). More highly fragmented embryos are given a lower grade and usually have worse implantation rates. Lower-grade embryos can be used or even improved using microsurgical fragment removal before embryo transfer. Studies suggest that those that implant successfully result in perfectly normal babies.

PGD, increasingly available at ART clinics, entails removing a single cell from an eight-cell embryo and analyzing its chromosomal composition using fluorescent in situ hybridization (FISH), giving embryologists, doctors, and patients the opportunity to test for genetic normalcy prior to transfer. Clinics compiling PGD data have found that 90 percent of embryos biopsied in women over forty are genetically abnormal. For a woman of thirty-five, the total risk for chromosomal abnormality as demonstrated by amniocentesis is 1 in 132; at age forty it is 1 in 51; and by age forty-five it increases to 1 in 12, a result of prolonged exposure to environmental mutagens. PGD has proven that some embryos that appear to be microscopically abnormal are actually genetically normal, while flawless-looking embryos may be abnormal. This fact helps explain the decreased fertility rates and increased rates of miscarriage and genetic abnormalities in older women.

PGD could dramatically reduce birth defects and increase pregnancy rates, no matter the patient's age, allowing doctors to transfer only normal and therefore theoretically viable embryos. It also gives objective information to patients who just can't get pregnant, even when their embryos look ideal under a microscope. If a majority of a patient's embryos tested as genetically abnormal, she might choose to use donor eggs from the get-go, sparing herself the disappointment and expense of repeated failed transfers. PGD could also help ease the knotty ethical dilemmas brought about when traditional tests such as amniocentesis or chorionic villus sampling turn up genetic abnormalities in a fetus.

Since no truly reliable way of reducing the incidence of multifetal pregnancies exists, some countries have adopted laws limiting how many embryos a doctor may transfer. The British maximum is two, while some Scandinavian clinics transfer only one embryo in younger patients. Doctors who violate the rules may lose their license, pay a fine, or face jail time. In the United States and India, where there are no laws prescribing how private fertility clinics conduct business, it's typical to transfer four embryos in younger patients and upward of six in older ones.

In 1971 the twin birth rate stood at about 1 in 60, while today it is closer to 1 in 30. The number of births involving three or more babies has quadrupled. Experts conclude that one-third of the increase can be attributed to the natural tendency for older moms to have twins, while fertility treatments account for the remaining two-thirds. Studies suggest that between 30 and 40 percent of pregnancies with three or more babies, aka "supertwins," are the result of IVF; fewer than one in five high-order multiple pregnancies result from natural conception.

In 2002 approximately 35 percent of IVF births in the United States were multiples, and 4 percent were triplets or more. In Finland and Sweden, where 60 percent of IVF procedures involve transferring only one embryo, the multiple-pregnancy rate has fallen to under 10 percent, with a triplet rate of zero. In 1999 the CDC reported that between 10 and 13 percent of women under thirty-five, the group most likely to get pregnant with multiples following IVF, who had three embryos transferred, ended up pregnant with triplets. The CDC also found that, for women with healthy eggs, placing three embryos yielded no higher a pregnancy rate than placing two. The ASRM, in 2002, issued voluntary guidelines recommending that women under thirty-five with a good prognosis should strongly consider placing only one embryo or, barring extraordinary circumstances, no more than two. Women between thirty-five and thirty-seven with a good prognosis should receive two embryos or, in more challenging medical circumstances, a maximum of three. But the guidelines, being voluntary, are not enforceable and often ignored.

In October 2005 *The Wall Street Journal* ran a story by Sylvia Pagán Westphal about the high incidence of IVF multiples. Clinics, said the story, bypass the ASRM guidelines and offer patients crowded transfers. Examining CDC records for 2002, the *Journal* found that 33 percent of clinics still place an average of more than three embryos in women younger than thirty-five. These clinics downplay the risk of multiples to their patients, pregnancy, no matter the degree, being their main concern. In one instance, clinicians assured a surrogate mother that the odds that a single embryo would take was only one in thirty. Based on such a dismal prognosis, she agreed to transfer five. Defying the odds, and helping the clinic's pregnancy rates, she became pregnant with quintuplets.

Doctors whom the *Journal* interviewed cite inferior embryo quality as a rationale for implanting more embryos than the ASRM guidelines suggest. Dr. Rifaat Salem of the Pacific Reproductive Center in Torrance, California, explains that he disregards the guidelines when treating a patient who has several failed attempts under her belt. He'll gladly place ten or twelve embryos in some women, he acknowledges, even those under thirty-five, if their embryos are of inferior quality. None of the patients who have had upward of ten embryos placed have given birth to high-order multiples, he claims, not offering whether any had selectively reduced a high-order multiple pregnancy.

According to the *Journal* article, Dr. Salem placed four embryos in one thirty-four-year-old patient, telling the patient and her husband that, due to inferior embryonic quality, this was their best course of treatment. The couple agreed to the populous transfer and ended up pregnant with quadruplets, a situation that, upon obstetric advice, was reduced by half. Pregnant with twins, the patient went into early labor and gave birth to severely premature infants. One of the twins, a girl, contracted a fungal infection and died at two months; her mother had held her only twice. The surviving twin, at almost two years old, still relies on a feeding tube. In the intervening years, Pacific began offering a chromosomal test to measure embryonic viability. The test is not perfect, as Dr. Patrizio's study bears out, but still it has caused Pacific to cut back on the average number of embryos transferred from a one-time high of 4.5 embryos in their younger patients.

I actually visited Pacific Reproductive Center when a good friend's wedding necessitated a mid-IVF trip to California. I planned a three-night stay, one in L.A. to see my dad and brother; then on to Marin for the wedding. It wasn't like I was headed to Mongolia, I told myself, my mother, and Gary; I was going to L.A., the red-hot center of the ART world, should I require any care. But why would I? Things were going well, I was still only at the stimulation portion of my cycle, and I'd be home in time for my next regularly scheduled monitoring appointment.

During the flight I felt sharp cramps and a terrible fullness. I went to the lavatory and was surprised at the obvious physical change since I left home that morning. I stood on the toilet console, hunched over, and examined my profile. Like the Incredible Hulk, or a liposuction success pictorial in reverse, my body had suddenly transformed: my abdomen was distended, and my belly button resembled the rolled latex knotting an overly inflated balloon.

When we landed, I called Dr. Hamlin's office. The nurse I spoke with consulted a list of ASRM-affiliated clinics in the L.A. area, gave me the number for Pacific Reproductive Center, and instructed me to mention that I was a patient of Dr. Hamlin's. The doctor who saw me the following morning (I don't think it was Salem) disapproved of my traveling during an IVF cycle but said everything looked fine and that my follicles were developing like gangbusters. He even asked if he could share my ultrasound image with a patient whom he was having difficulty stimulating. I didn't know how she'd profit by seeing the image, and it seemed callous to flaunt somebody else's abundance; egg stimulation was his job, not hers. Even so, I agreed.

By the time we got to the Bay Area, I was even more bloated, attracting the approving looks that pregnant women get from strangers. I had begun vomiting and strained to catch my breath. Once more I called Dr. Hamlin, who arranged for me to visit a clinic run by a former colleague. The doctor who examined me said I was experiencing ovarian hyperstimulating syndrome (OHSS), the most serious complication of IVF. He explained that my polycystic ovaries put me at risk for it, as did my relatively young age. My ovaries were so swollen, he said, as to require putting an end to the cycle posthaste. He hooked me up to an IV to restore my fluids and electrolyte balance, told me to drink plenty of Gatorade over the next couple of days, and explained that if I continued taking the follicle-stimulating drugs or if I moved around jerkily, I'd be at serious risk of an ovary twist. An ovary that twists upon itself cuts off its own blood supply, which can lead to death of the tissue, gangrene, and amputation.

"I'll call your doctor, Hamlin, and explain my findings and recommendation."

"Would Dr. Hamlin have another plan? You know, an alternative to scrapping the cycle?"

"Not if he's competent, he wouldn't," the doctor said, telling me to enjoy my friend's wedding, and exited the exam room.

The Wall Street Journal reports that fertility clinics control their patient population to improve overall success rates. They refuse to treat older patients or those whose medical histories counterindicate pregnancy. They also test potential patients before admitting them into their programs. For example, if a patient does not produce eggs in response to hormone shots, she's rejected so she won't negatively impact the clinic's numbers. Clinics also, as reported in the media and recounted anecdotally by people I know, lowball a woman's odds at success, convincing her that populous transfers are in the best interest of achieving a pregnancy.

But clinicians say that patients, adamant in their desire for pregnancy, can be aggressive. Often they've put aside a career to pursue it, temporarily moved to be near a particular clinic, borrowed money or refinanced their home, and they resent, or downright reject, any limits placed on their treatment. I know women who admit to pressuring their doctors, begging them to be aggressive when it comes to numbers of embryos, not wanting caution to cost them their baby. They assure everyone involved—their medical team, their partners, themselves—

that they'll make responsible, reasoned choices once they've achieved pregnancy. By the time a woman is at the point of transfer, she's typically been through the wringer or has babies on the brain, and feels desperate or is otherwise incapable of making an informed, rational decision as to whether to transfer more than two embryos or to play it safe, multiples-wise, and ask for the single best-looking one. So she goes for broke.

Plenty of doctors are more than willing to comply, knowing that statistics are being kept and success rates tallied and made public by the CDC. Fertility clinics, competing for patients, advertise in newspapers, magazines, and on TV. They aggressively market patient-friendly financial arrangements, increasingly offering payment option choices. A patient can choose an à la carte program, paying $7,500 per attempt regardless of the outcome. Or she can choose a money-back guarantee and pay $15,000, which covers up to three attempts with the promise that if no live birth delivery occurs, the full $15,000 will be refunded. Since clinics are hardly charities, one wonders how it is they can make such offers and still remain profitable. The answer might be that such arrangements bring in younger and less infertile patients, inducing people who might otherwise successfully employ less invasive procedures, with fewer side effects and lower risks of multiple births, to try IVF first.

Knowing that potential patients comparison-shop, ART clinics work hard to distinguish themselves in the marketplace. They hire specialty marketing firms with confidence-inducing names like FemPartners and IntegraMed to increase their visibility and patient rosters. They craft elaborate websites with long, orderly lists of all they can provide, the squads of fertility professionals at their patients' disposal, and photos like airbrushed publicity shots of the embryos they've created.

Conception has emerged as a frequent cultural topic. Stories on embryo transfers gone wrong, high-order multiple births, and older women having babies are everywhere. Newspapers and magazines run full-page ads seeking egg donors and infertile patients. Gender-determination tests for pregnant women are featured as human interest stories on local newscasts. Regional clinics advertise on daytime TV, highlighting money-back guarantees and hand-holding couples brought closer through their travails. In the early 1970s, when assisted reproductive treatments first became available, infertility was a taboo topic. People were embarrassed to discuss it, and if they sought treatment, they did so discreetly. But in this day and age of direct-to-consumer medication marketing, of jackhammer-wielding toe fungi and allergy mascots with a shape and color suggestive of boogers, an attractive couple discussing their infertility no longer seems so unmentionable.

In August 2005 *conceive magazine* debuted, and always with a glossy cover photo of a baby with skin like yeasty dough and pin-lit eyes. It features "stories of women who have achieved their dream of parenthood," pieces on fertility diets and how to avoid conception burnout. *conceive* has trademarked the phrases "America's first fertility magazine" and "celebrating the creation of families," its very existence and critical success demonstrating that bearing children is not only a commercial enterprise but also, with its often arduous trek and sometimes breathtaking results, as dramatic as the Iditarod.

Taking the opposite titular tack, *Inconceivable* was a short-lived drama on NBC that premiered on September 23, 2005, and had its series finale on September 30, 2005. It was described by NBC thusly:

> This delightful ensemble drama concerns one of the most complicated questions: to conceive or not to conceive. The doctors of the Family Options Fertility Clinic are on a noble quest to help desperate couples give birth. Except these doctors are often distracted by their personal quests involving

sex, deception and secrets. Navigating through ultrasounds and superegos, missing frozen embryos and impending malpractice suits, it's positively clear that life inside this clinic is anything but sterile.

Having tuned in for the show's entire season (I want my two hours back), I must assume that *delightful* is a euphemism for *inane*. But like any melodrama, with its exaggerated take on how people live (and its population of ultrasexy and OSHA-violatingly shod clinicians), it was entertaining. This was a terrible clinic, perhaps the world's worst, run by a doctor whose semen actually infiltrated a patient's supply. Certainly real-world clinics make mistakes, as the white British couple who underwent IVF and gave birth to black twins discovered, as did the Dutch fraternal brothers, one black and one white. But a reproductive specialist getting fellated by a spurned lab technician who agilely transfers the doctor's genetic stuff from her mouth to a vial and switches a label or two—that's just not the sort of activity the ASRM wants its affiliate members engaging in.

The potential market, and the potential for profit, is huge. According to the National Center for Health Statistics (NCHS), a health-monitoring organization under the auspices of the CDC, more than a million women report having medical infertility consultations each year, and the number of women aged fifteen to forty-four with an impaired ability to have children exceeds six million. More than nine million women have used infertility services, and approximately 300,000 are undergoing treatment at any given time. More than two million married couples are considered infertile. Fertility specialists, and the media, have responded by upping their offerings and giving interested constituencies what they think they want, for better or worse.

Certainly plenty of ART professionals worry more about the

health of their patients and their potential children than about ticks on a success rate chart. They follow professional guidelines and require their patients to respect clinic protocol, no matter who's footing the bill. They medicate conservatively, transfer the minimum number of embryos possible, and advise their patients to "take the path of least regret," admonishing them to thoroughly consider every decision and, once the embryos have been transferred, not to do anything that might later stand out as the reason a cycle failed.

But lacking a formal medical education and already having put instinct way aside, I never quite knew where this path lay. I recognized obvious pitfalls—dead lifting, fasting, and gangbangs—activities I routinely avoided anyway. But how could I be sure that pumping gas hadn't sent pregnancy-impeding fumes through my body? Or that watching emotional TV dramas—like an episode of *ER* that featured a pregnant mother in a car wreck, surviving even as her baby was stillborn—wouldn't cause my body to pump adrenaline that'd wreck my own pregnancy? Bickering with my mother or picking up after my dog; braving traffic on my way to school and, once there, soaking in whatever toxins the fluorescent lights and copy machines emitted in the asbestos-insulated, lead-painted eighty-year-old building; would these be harmful? In other words, I never quite knew which of the several activities constituting my everyday routine might ultimately stand out as regrettable.

My first successful round of IVF occurred three years shy of the ASRM recommended age. I was thirty-one and Dr. Hamlin transferred three textbook-perfect, blastocyst-stage embryos. But I'd conceived only one child, Sophia.

By every measure I'd been a candidate for replacing only a limited number of embryos, and even though I understood the lack of embryonic predictability and the medical dilemmas precipitated by it, if the clinic had tried to limit my embryo replacement, I most likely would have objected. So what, I would have argued, if I get pregnant with triplets? That'd be wonderful, the best possible outcome. It'd save us time and money, and what's so scary about triplets anyway? People have them left and right (and left again) these days. And so what if they arrived a little early? Northwestern Memorial, our hospital of choice, had a Level III neonatal intensive care unit (NICU). That is, if their kick-ass team of high-risk perinatologists couldn't nurse me to the end of my full gestational term.

I know women who, opposed to selective reduction and eager for one baby at a time, chose to transfer a single embryo per round. A few got lucky (or benefited from God's grace or the embryologist's discerning eye) and ended up pregnant. More often they didn't succeed, at least not on the first try. Some of them stuck to their guns, pacing their IVF to prevent a multiple pregnancy. But for the more ambivalent and less patient among us, this was an excruciating decision to have to make.

I imagine myself in two years, surrounded by shirtless and food-splattered quintuplets bawling in dirty-diapered heaps about the unmopped kitchen floor, lists of tutors and physical therapists taped to the fridge I am excavating in search of something unrancid enough to eat. Or in twenty years on a Caribbean cruise for voluntarily childless couples. Dressed in a sparkly gown, skin tough and splotchy as a desert iguana's from all the vacations we've had time to take, we dine with a group of similarly unencumbered people, and I drink too much, as usual, and start crying, letting my head flop on the shoulder of the tuxedoed dude next to me, gushing that I'm not voluntarily childless, that we are cruising under false pretenses. He squeezes my knee and reassures me that the world is an oyster and that children prevent one from slurping it down. And anyway, he continues, the world is much too scary a place to raise kids in.

All I know is that I want to get pregnant and hope the announcement will carry a wallop. Most dramatic would be triplets. But twins would make for exciting phone calls to our family and friends, too. When Debbie advises that I am sitting on very strong embryos, and that transferring three, the maximum they allow, will likely result in multiples, I urge her to load 'em up. Gary, confident that I can act decisively if faced with a lifeboat situation and will agree to follow medical advice if counseled to reduce a risky pregnancy, concurs. But after Debbie leaves, I confess that I don't know how people selectively reduce their pregnancies.

"I mean, it's still an abortion," I say. "And it's not like we'd be using it to deal with an unwanted or unintended pregnancy, even if that were justification enough. We've labored and sacrificed to create whatever fetus results. And barring a terrible birth defect, I just can't imagine reducing the pregnancy as if it were any other tool in the ART cache, like all the other production methods. I mean, could you agree to sacrificing a baby that you'd so, so, so intentionally created?"

"If a doctor advised it, you betcha," Gary says.

"It just seems monstrous to strive for something, to work and pray for its development, and then to purge it when it no longer seems like the best result."

"But you just said you would," he says, "to Debbie. And more importantly, to me."

"I know I did. And I would. I mean, if I had to. But I think it'd haunt me forever. Possibly drive me crazy."

"I'm finding Debbie and telling her we'll just take the best one," Gary says, sliding the alcove curtain to the side. "We can't risk it, not with your indecision."

"Don't you dare!" I say, "Listen, we enlisted medicine to get this far, and I promise to use it to the end. If I need to take action, even ugly and possibly sinful action, trust me, I'll agree to it."

Truth is, while going through IVF, my views on abortion had shifted. At one time, I considered it a practical matter, a solution for an unintended or unwanted pregnancy, no matter the circumstances. But as I struggled to achieve pregnancy and thought deeply and often about the intangibility, unpredictability, and blessing of life, my consciousness changed. I could no longer view it in purely political terms or as a simple matter of choice.

I know plenty of people who have had abortions. Some of them did so after finding out that a gestating baby had a significant disability, and still struggled with the decision. But most had an abortion because the timing of the pregnancy didn't feel right, or because they didn't want to marry the baby's father and didn't want to raise it alone. But what of these babies that Gary and I have wanted nothing more than to create? I mean, I haven't undergone IVF with a specific end in mind, one boy, or a mixed set of twins. I haven't cared if I had one or four at a time, and I've been more than willing to see even an inconvenient result through.

Unlike the right-to-lifers I had once faced down at abortion rights rallies, the chanting crowd on one side of the issue, my side of the issue, wielding hand-painted NO TRESPASSING IN MY UTERUS signs, while those on the other side flaunted humongous photos of aborted fetuses, I understood the many legitimate reasons to keep abortion accessible, safe, and legal, not least among them the importance of a woman retaining control over her own body. But my recent exposure to the science behind creating life, the knowledge of how early the heart is formed, how soon it begins to beat, forced upon me a new perspective. I haven't suddenly embraced fetal legal rights, nor do I think a fetus should actually be countable on a census. But experiencing IVF has taught me how profound this choice is and that what's at stake extends far beyond exercising one's rights or minimizing one's complications.

Certainly embryo reductions are often performed for medically legitimate reasons. Multifetal pregnancies carry a high risk of premature birth. Babies born at 22 weeks or earlier have little chance of surviving. Babies born between 23 and 24 weeks increase their survival rate by 3 to 4 percent per day, those between 24 and 26 weeks survive at rates of 20 to 30 percent. Survival for preemies after 26 weeks is as high as 60 to 90 percent, depending on the baby's condition at time of delivery and how much he or she improves with medical care. But preemies are born with immature and incompletely developed parts, most notably their brains. Disproportionate numbers of learning disabilities and psychiatric illness occur in people who are born prematurely.

A January 2005 study from the Queen's Medical Centre in Nottingham, England, considered 241 six-year-olds who had all been born three months premature. While only about 10 percent had significant physical disabilities, over 40 percent had learning difficulties, more than had been predicted. In the United States, one in five premature kids ends up repeating at least one grade. A July 20, 2005, study published in the *Journal of the American Medical Association* looked at eight-year-olds who had weighed less than 2.2 pounds at birth (extremely low birth-weight, or ELBW, children). These ELBW children were more likely than their full-term counterparts to have considerable long-term health and educational needs, lower IQs, and inferior academic and motor skills. These children "fared substantially worse than [normal birth-weight children] in every type of assessment," said the article. The final paragraph summed up the dire situation, one that has been created, in large part, by the improvement in technologies to keep these tiniest of babies alive in the NICU:

> In the United States in 2002, there were 22,845 live births with a birth weight of 500 to 999 g, of whom approximately 70% survived. Our findings underscore the extraordinary costs of care that will be needed to manage the medical, educational, and other service needs of the large proportion of these ELBW children who develop chronic conditions . . . The American Academy of Pediatrics has emphasized the importance of providing a medical home for children with special health care needs, coordinating their care, involving

family, and assisting in navigation of the complex federal, state, and local systems that provide services required by these children. All of these services are highly relevant for the continuing long-term care of ELBW children who survive as a result of neonatal intensive care.

But statistics and studies aside, all these years later I'm still wondering at what point the embryos that didn't take hold folded. I'm still wondering whether I mindlessly flushed them or if my body absorbed them silently, invisibly, while I was mentally decorating the nursery. I also still wonder whether, like the stretch marks remaining from pregnancy, the disappeared embryos are now a permanent part of my physical makeup, an extra few cells on my bladder walls, or, as I like to think, residing somewhere in my heart.

Prematurity is correlated with gestational diabetes, preeclampsia, and infant mortality. Improved antenatal technologies are giving obstetricians the chance to assess fetal well-being and to diagnose fetal compromise in previously unavailable ways. But, like assisted reproductive technologies, these diagnostic capabilities generate their own ethical dilemmas. Say there are twins, one of whom thrives in utero while his co-twin struggles. Does a person—a parent or doctor—put the healthy twin at risk from preterm delivery to treat the compromised one? Or is it somehow more ethical to allow the compromised twin to perish in utero in order to buy crucial gestational time for the healthy twin?

I went through IVF early enough to dodge the ASRM guidelines, a personal boon despite the legitimate problems they address. In the first place, limits give people who would never consider selective reduction an option, lending them an inalterable rationale for not transferring all the existing embryos and, in the process, sparing them the moral dilemma surrounding a high-order multiple pregnancy—whether to do nothing and knowingly expose the high-order multiples to grave risk, or rather to undergo a prophylactic procedure that they know is not only forbidden, but the very peak of sin mountain.

Secondly, for impetuous folks or those who don't fully appreciate the risk, an administrative rule would protect them, and their children, from a naïve gamble. Limits would certainly help check the present-day explosion in multiple births. In my neck of the woods I see them almost daily, the Escalade-like stretch triplet strollers occupied by look-alike kids in identical hats being pushed by shivering nannies from tropical countries, wending their cumbersome way over sidewalks, slush, and minimountains of plowed snow. Here in my largely affluent suburban Chicago town, most of these young multiples are very likely the result of one fertility treatment or another. When Gary and I (or our nanny) go out with our kids, people probably come to the same, accurate conclusion about us.

When the twins were still babies and more clearly the same age (Lily now has a good dozen pounds on Anna), we'd walk down our shady Lincoln Park street, Anna and Lily suspended from our chests in BabyBjörn baby carriers, their snowsuited arms and legs sticking stiffly through the holes. I'd push Sophia's tastefully plaid Italian stroller while Gary held tight to the matching collar and leash adorning Phoebe, our pure-bred dog. People would look at us, grin, and comment on our pack. "You must have your hands full," they'd say, almost to a person. I'd smile and tell them they were right, our hands were full, sometimes adding a wish for octopus parts. I'd watch to see if they'd scan us for other signs of riches—a pair of shoes I'd indulged in, say, or an expensive wristwatch. Or were our kids, our dog, our only excesses?

In fact, our kids were not our only luxury. Once we had them and could no longer travel or go out to restaurants or parties or movies or anywhere else without making elaborate arrangements, I found other avenues for splurging: organic

produce and Grey Goose vodka, smocked dresses and baby en-
richment classes. Their technological beginnings also sparked
a reactionary impulse in me. After all that time I'd spent ceding natural processes to doctors and technology, I pursued being an Earth Mother (with a taste for good booze) rather than
a technologically enabled one. I dragged out my old Grateful
Dead T-shirts and wore them with recycled cotton pants ripped
at the knees, Birkenstocks, and socks woven from hemp. I
steamed brown rice for dinner, bought farm-raised meats, and
prepared my own baby food, boiling the yams and mashing
them with a make-your-own-baby-food contraption that my
Los Angeles stepmother sent me along with child psychology
books. I nursed the girls (pumping and dumping the first
round to limit how much vodka and Pinot they'd end up with)
and wore them in batiked slings like bulky bandoliers.

Only the shirts were decades old and falling apart, so I returned them to the box I took them from, the one also containing my high school cheerleading skirt and vest, my Camp
Birch Trail T-shirts, my hard hat and riding crop from when I
was certain I'd be a professional horseback rider, and my pre-
teen diary with the broken lock on the side. Likewise the cotton pants that ripped a little more each time I wore them, my
knees sticking out the fronts like rising dough. The girls didn't
especially like the food I boiled and mashed, and it was so
much easier just to buy the premade stuff in the jars with the
label showing a hippie baby—how else to explain the lack of
clothing, the sunburned face, the alfalfa patch for a play-
ground? I also stopped nursing the twins once they hit seven
months and their heads got too large for me to accommodate
both drinkers at one time-efficient time.

I found out I was having twins at five weeks, when the ultrasound plainly showed two separate sacs, two beating hearts. I
was simultaneously elated and anxious. I worried about the
hard work of the pregnancy, the first few months and years, the

psychological and physical issues our kids might face by virtue of their twinship, and how Sophia would fare when faced with attention-grabbing and perhaps hair-pulling twin siblings. But I was thrilled about the efficiency of it all. We'd have two babies for the price of one round of IVF—three children with only two pregnancies—and kids close enough in age that we'd be able to choose fewer activities to satisfy all their needs. There'd be fewer toys, fewer clothes, fewer play dates, and one less birthday party to plan and execute.

The twin pregnancy seemed to be progressing so smoothly, as the first had, that I was seeing one of my regular doctor's partners. At the twenty-first gestational week, however, it went seriously south. I went in for a routine obstetrical check, and a few seconds into the internal exam, the doctor informed me, by way of those extraordinarily telling syllables *uh* and *oh*, that she didn't like what she felt. Rotating her arm one way and swiveling her hand back in the other direction, she bowed her head and closed her eyes in sheer concentration. Looking back up at me, she removed her hand, pulled the sheet back over my legs, peeled off her glove, and told me to sit up.

She was able to fit two of her fingers inside my cervix, she reported, a sign that it had weakened. Even at twenty-one weeks, when the twins' combined weight couldn't have been more than a pound and a half, my cervix was failing under the pressure. One of the major causes of miscarriage, she explained, is incompetent cervix, and it seemed that that was where I was headed. I wasn't contracting, however, and she said that was a blessing. But I should plan on going to the hospital, and she asked what else, besides ordering a wheelchair and getting my charts ready, she could do for me.

The office was a couple of short blocks from Northwestern's Prentice Women's Hospital, where I was wheeled and admitted. An en route call to Gary let him know he should meet me there on the double. I was taken to a labor and delivery room a couple doors down from where I had Sophia and was told to change into a hospital gown. Dr. Golden had been paged and, just finishing a delivery right down the hall, rushed in and asked me what was going on. She examined me, concurred with her partner's assessment, and enumerated our options.

We could do nothing, a choice that almost certainly meant we'd lose the pregnancy. If that was our wish, to let nature take its course, Dr. Golden said, she'd stick around and deliver the doomed babies for us. Or we could try to stem the dilation by placing a cervical cerclage, a band of strong thread woven around the cervix and pulled to close and tighten it. Yes, I said, confused that that hadn't been offered up as course of treatment number one and noting how beautiful a word it was. *Cerclage. Cerclage*, like a dance or a dressmaking technique. Of course, let's do a cerclage!

Problem was, Dr. Golden explained, a cerclage usually bought only two to three weeks, and our babies needed much more than that even to survive. Let's say we went ahead, put in the stitch, and made it to twenty-four weeks, the age of viability, our children would most likely face severe troubles. Golden ticked off a few, using her fingers to represent the various catastrophes. Blindness. Deafness. Cerebral palsy. Mental retardation. She held up her pinkie and said, "That is, if they even survive."

The procedure itself also carried risks, including uterine or bladder rupture, maternal hemorrhage, cervical infection, preterm labor, premature rupture of the membranes, and the potential for cervical laceration if I went into labor with the stitch still in place. If our pregnancy weren't so highly invested, she said (meaning if it had been naturally occurring), she'd most likely advise against a cerclage at such a precarious gestational moment. But she understood that it was no ordinary pregnancy, it was a so-called "premium pregnancy," and that achieving it again could not be taken for granted. She also had enormous faith in a particular surgeon, a Dr. Rob Graff. She phoned him and confirmed that he could operate later that evening.

Before consenting to the surgery, Gary and I extracted a promise from Dr. Golden, and each other, that we'd not push to save the babies, to employ any drastic life-saving measures, if they arrived even a minute before their twenty-fourth week. It was a devastating thing to have to decide, even to have to consider. But it was the only way I could go through with it. I needed to be a realist, and realistically, I couldn't stand the thought of these tiny translucent children born too soon, hooked up to machinery and sealed off from the viral world in plastic incubators, the potential for death from infection at a few weeks of age, or a life spent attached to tubes and monitors striking me as too selfish and cruel not to address and plot against.

The anesthesiologist entered the room, a paper mask dangling at his neck. I recognized him as the handsome guy who had done my epidural when I had Sophia. Clearly not remembering me (perhaps my sway back, the one he commented on as a professional challenge, would jog his memory), he introduced himself and said he was going to do an epidural and did I have any questions about the procedure.

"I had an epidural when I gave birth to my daughter," I told him. "I guess that means I generally know what to expect. Except I really shook a lot last time, as it wore off."

"That's a fairly common side effect," he said. "You know, it's a relief that you already have a kid. That should really take the pressure off this one. How long since you last ate?"

"It's twins," Gary said. "And no, we don't feel relaxed in the least. This is terrible, and everybody here needs to treat it as a major crisis. Okay?"

"No offense, buddy," the anesthesiologist said. I loved Gary for standing up for our babies and what I was going through, but I hoped he hadn't offended the man about to pop a tube into my spinal column.

"I ate a spinach croissant from the coffee shop where Dr. Golden's office is right before my checkup, so I guess that was, what, five and a half, six hours ago?"

The anesthesiologist said that was fine, sounded yummy, handed me a pillow, instructed me to lean forward over it and to stay perfectly still. "I'll use an iodine solution to sterilize the site," he said. "It'll feel cold." He told me to take a deep breath and hold it while he placed the needle between two of my vertebrae and threaded the fine medication-delivering tube through it and into the epidural space that lies between the outermost covering of the spinal cord and the vertebral canal formed by the spine bones. I felt a burning beneath my skin, something I hadn't noticed when laboring with Sophia, what with all the crowding at my pain receptors. Within a couple of minutes, sensation below my waist was blocked, and I was being introduced to Dr. Graff.

Dr. Graff had been one of Dr. Golden's interns, or something like that, and they were delighted to see each other. They kissed and hugged and inquired about children and mutual friends and colleagues, this while I feared a yawning cervix, this while Gary fought back panic.

"You couldn't be in better hands," Dr. Golden said to me and Gary, by way of reassuring us and of complimenting her former student. "Rob is not only the nicest guy around, he is an incredibly capable surgeon."

She explained the current situation to Dr. Graff, noting that she hadn't detected any further dilation. Upon her last examination, she said, I was at around two and a half centimeters. (Once you've dilated four centimeters, the procedure is no longer effective or even an option.) I understood the real risk that the cerclage might not hold, she continued, apprising Graff but looking at me. Nevertheless, I had agreed to try it and had already received my epidural.

"Sounds fair," Dr. Graff said. He shook my hand and Gary's hand and told us he'd see us in a few minutes.

I was wheeled into an operating room and transferred to a table with stirrups projecting off the end, like the one they used at Great Lakes. I shivered as Dr. Golden positioned the light. "A little pressure," she said as she put in a speculum (probably out of habit since I could feel nothing) and proceeded to clean my cervix, again with an iodine solution. Dr. Graff came over and examined me. Looking up at the metallic overhead light, I caught a reflection of giant, purple-stained cotton swabs on the table and of the doctors working between my splayed legs.

While Dr. Graff checked my cervix, Dr. Golden explained that she'd been able to insert two-plus fingers. Dr. Graff said he thought it might be even more than that, closer to three-plus of his larger fingers, a figure he converted to centimeters, like the talk at the back of a geeky school's bus or the boasting in the green room at a chess championship.

Graff worked for about an hour. He pulled at the thread as if he were quilting and finally tugged the ends to resecure my cervix.

"Perfect. All set," he said. "It's completely closed."

"Do you think it'll hold until Beth gets to a safe enough point to have the babies?" Gary asked. "I mean, Dr. Golden explained everything, but do you think maybe it isn't as bad as we thought before the surgery?"

"As long as no contractions tug at the stitch," he said, "it should hold. But I'm sure Dr. Golden explained that all this messing around we've done down there can sometimes stir things up and provoke contractions."

To that end, I was monitored throughout the night. Based on my uterine peace and cervical stability, I was sent home the following morning and ordered on strict bed rest. I was to lie in bed all day, every day. I was to be not entirely supine, since my pregnant and heavy belly would put too much pressure on my internal organs, but I was definitely not to sit upright either, since that would impact my cervix. I was to eat my meals in bed in a semiprone position, elevated only as much as absolutely necessary to avoid choking. A seated shower every other day, trips to the bathroom, and occasional cab rides to the doctor were the only allowable activities. Gary bought a tray upon which to carry meals to me, added a few magazines to our subscription list, brought home novels and biographies, and upped the babysitter's hours for one-and-a-half-year-old Sophia, who, proving herself an unreformable bed-jumper, was basically banished from our room unless escorted by her father.

Statistically, up to 700,000 expectant women a year, or one in five moms-to-be, are prescribed bed rest during complicated pregnancies, yet there is no hard and fast science proving its benefits. Aerospace scientists who have studied its side effects (the effects of bed rest and space flight, two weightless activities, are nearly identical) find that bed rest causes musculoskeletal, cardiovascular, and psychological problems. Judith A. Maloni, Ph.D., R.N., and author of *Antepartum Bed Rest: Case Studies, Research, and Nursing Care*, wrote a report on the aerospace studies called "Astronauts and Bed Rest: What NASA is teaching us about inactivity . . ." On its cover a pregnant woman beams. She rests comfortably inside a space capsule, the rounded orb of her inhabited belly eclipsing the bright light of the sun shining on its nonvisible, southern exposure.

According to Maloni, in the early 1940s NASA and other aerospace scientists began putting people on bed rest to study the potential effects of weightlessness in space. Five-ish decades of research later they have determined that bed rest effects change in every bodily system. Based on these findings, in fact, nonpregnant patients were encouraged to get out of bed and move around to promote recovery, particularly after surgery.

The NASA study showed rapid and negative physical adaptation to a prolonged horizontal state. For example, bodily flu-

ids shift from the feet toward the head, increasing urine production (diuresis) to rid the body of excess fluids in the chest
and head. Baroreceptors located in the chest that help regulate
blood pressure as posture shifts no longer get stimulated, resulting in low blood pressure, and dizziness or fainting, when a
person stands up (orthostatic hypotension). Muscles weaken
and atrophy, and bones deteriorate within twenty-four to forty-
eight hours. The body's loss of postural cues stimulates change
in circadian rhythms, resulting in abnormal sleep patterns during immobility, leading to fatigue. Astronauts on space missions
and pregnant women on bed rest also experience weight loss or
slow weight gain, headache, and indigestion.

The researchers determined that pregnancy bed rest and
space flight can alter psychological states. Both are commonly
accompanied by feelings of estrangement from the familiar,
an enforced and insurmountable separation from friends and
family, and a sense of confinement, boredom, and depression
arising from ongoing sensory deprivation. Maloni's report not
only catalogues the problems but also offers up some helpful
coping tips. For one, small frequent meals and raising the head
of the bed will help with indigestion. Also, putting on some
makeup and fixing your hair as you normally would, even if
you'll be the only one to see you all day, and even if somebody
else will have to remove the rouge and lipstick stains from
your bedding, is seen as an effective and easy way to stave off
depression.

As a woman who now has healthy babies to show for her
risky, nearly tragic pregnancy, I don't ultimately care if bed rest
is controversial, whether it was a waste of my time or my inner
resources or our babysitting dollars or the goodwill of my insurance company. I went from dangerously close to losing the
girls to having them at a relatively safe gestational age. My bed
rest wasn't easy, particularly since it began on September 14,
2001, three days after the terrorist attacks. I spent way too many
hours watching the footage, ignoring the expert warnings not

to view the images too many times for fear of permanent psychological damage. I also pined for Sophia. I hated sending her to mother-child bonding classes with a babysitter. I hated missing several of her "firsts"—her first full grammatical sentence, first pepperoni, that kind of thing. But my enforced confinement, and my constant fear that I'd wake up in a puddle containing their lifeblood, have endowed me with total appreciation for my kids and a fairly complete satisfaction just being with them, no matter the otherwise mind-numbing circumstances. And that, NASA be damned, is good enough for me.

Some women are hospitalized for their bed rest, as I finally was when my contractions proved out of control. They're monitored at regular intervals, have ultrasounds several times a day, and are examined by different doctors rounding on different schedules. If they're at a teaching hospital—a wonderful institution conceptually but an often hilariously frustrating one in cervix exhibiting theory—they get to help medical students expand their body of knowledge. Many women's hospitals have entire antenatal floors, with occupants at various levels of dire need, their beds at various states of recline, with the most severe cases—the women whose doctors have determined to keep all pressure off their cervixes—forced to rest with their hips and legs tipped 15 to 18 degrees higher than their shoulders in what is called the Trendelenburg position.

All told, my bed rest (and the remainder of my pregnancy) lasted fourteen weeks. I kept a notebook next to the bed to record my contractions, and whenever I had more than six in an hour, I knew the babies were in danger. At that point I'd be taken to labor and delivery, whisked to a room, and hooked up to an IV drip of magnesium sulfate, a tocolytic medication that slows uterine contractions during preterm labor. Magnesium is thought to affect the action of calcium in the body, and without sufficient calcium, uterine muscles cannot contract. It's the main ingredient in Epsom salts.

Each magnesium dose lasted until I was contraction-free for twenty-four hours. I had three doses. During those long periods I'd drift in and out of consciousness, mostly throwing up while awake—a somewhat common reaction to being "magged," as the nurses so dashingly called it. The nurses, Gary, and my mom, who drove in from Wisconsin to be with me and take care of Sophia, urged me to try to stop getting sick, to take deep breaths, and to think nonnauseating thoughts, concerned that the vomiting would squeeze my reactive uterus and spark new waves of contractions or tear my cerclage. Dr. Golden, upon being questioned about the pathetic shape of her patient and couldn't we just remove the IV, reminded us all that as bad as I clearly felt, it was nothing compared with how we'd all feel if we didn't take these aggressive measures to stem the contractions.

"But, Dr. Golden," I asked, my voice ricocheting around the kidney-shaped, bisque-colored plastic pan beneath my volatile mouth, "what is the magnesium's fetal impact?"

She assured me that the risks of prematurity far outweighed any risk of magnesium exposure. "I can't promise zero complications. But as long as those babies stay inside you, they'll stand a chance," she said. A study a year later in the *American Journal of Obstetrics and Gynecology* concluded, however, that infants whose mothers were given the drug were more than three times as likely to suffer from cerebral palsy, even when researchers accounted for other contributing factors.

In 2000 *Obstetrics and Gynecology* published the results of a study examining the link between perinatal death and tocolytic magnesium sulfate. The subjects included fetuses and "neonates" (newborns) who weighed between 700 and 1,249 grams (1.5 to 2.75 pounds) and found that exposure at a somewhat common dosage (48 grams or around 1.7 ounces) was "significantly associated with increased perinatal mortality." Intravenous magnesium can also accumulate in the body.

That is, if it isn't exiting regularly through urination or if the dosing isn't right, it can affect the maternal and fetal central nervous systems, impeding muscle control and breathing. It can also slow heartbeat and elevate the mother's blood pressure. If it got to that point, we would have no choice but to cease medication and let the contractions lead where they might.

Being on the floor where babies were delivered was also difficult, especially for Gary, who, going in and out of the room, encountered excited and proud new dads keen on questioning fellow presumed dads-to-be about their wives or partners, their new sons or daughters. Outside my door I'd hear the laboring women scream and whimper, their contractions traceable in their up-and-down moans. I'd hear crying newborns and families yelling out genders and names. "It's a girl! Maeve!" Or "A healthy baby boy! Jaden!" I'd also hear Gary asking the nurses if that mess lying atop a bedpan, the self-possessed woman he had married, was really okay. Had they taken my blood pressure lately? Had they asked me to squeeze their hands to make sure my muscles still worked?

My outcome was good. Fantastic, really, considering the risks we faced. The twins were born at thirty-five weeks. At over four pounds each, they were Amazonian by preemie standards. Only Lily, the younger by two minutes, who swallowed fluid during her feet-first exit, required any sort of stay in the NICU and, at two weeks, a relatively short one at that. Anna, though tiny, the flesh on her legs oversized and slack, like an elephant's skin or MC Hammer's pants, came home two days after being born, like any normal newborn. I actually wanted her to stay, not only so the girls could be in one place to maximize my time with both of them but to keep Lily company. It seemed wrong to separate them like this when Lily could really use the familiarity of her sister's heel in her ribs and elbow in her neck, the rhythm of her beating heart.

Among Lily's NICU-mates were other multiples, a few sets of preterm twins and triplets. I asked one of the nurses whether she thought they saw more multiples in the NICU these days, or was it just that so many multiples came early and had always ended up in there anyway? She said it was an interesting question, one she hadn't considered, and that she'd get back to me.

A few days later, at the scrub sink outside the NICU, I bumped into that nurse. She said she'd given my question some thought and wasn't sure whether the total numbers had changed, only the sorts of people who visited the babies. "For instance, you seem kind of young to be releasing more than one egg a month, which, as you might know, is why older ladies have a lot of the twins."

"Thank you," I said. She looked at me, confused. "For saying I look young."

"I'm just making a point," she said. "It used to be we had a lot of African American babies in here. And I may be wrong about this, but just from my experience, I'd have to guess that twins occur more frequently in that population. We still get them. But I'd say Caucasian and Indian twins are way up. We don't see many Asian ones. In my culture"—she was Filipino—"twins are seen as very bad luck. And using technological means to produce them is even worse. Very unnatural and untraditional. I guess the fact that those babies end up down here so often is proof of that."

I endeavored to spend my time at the NICU wisely, asking the nurses as many questions as I could about caring for premature infants. They showed me how to check to make sure Lily was eating sufficient amounts, how to keep her awake for feedings, how to promote both health and the mother-child bond using what they called "kangaroo care," whereby I would strip Lily down to her diaper and hat (and the monitor wires taped to her belly and feet) and slip her inside my blouse. I'd recline in a chair and sing to her, tell her stories, read the paper out loud, or nap.

I also asked after some of the other babies, particularly the ones I never saw anybody visit. Only the nurses would occasionally lift them out of their isolettes (the Frenchified and gussied-up term for the domed plastic incubators with holes on the sides for manual access, and casters on the bottom, like an airline serving cart or a steam table) and carry them around as they looked in on the others, filled out charts, and restocked formula or the stacks of minuscule, specialty diapers. The nurses said it was quite possible that these babies had been abandoned. Preemies and sick babies and others going through drug withdrawal are abandoned fairly frequently, they told me.

"It's very expensive to take care of sick babies," one of them explained. "Too much for some folks to handle. Some people can't stand to see their children like this, especially the parents whose behavior, their drugs or whatever, caused the problems in the first place. Some of the parents are just children themselves and lack the strength to deal with so big a problem. We do see our fair share of very responsible young mothers, but the thing I don't get is why a person, I don't care who they are, why she wouldn't at least turn the baby over to an adoption agency or a church, or even to a relative or a kind neighbor. There are so many people with big hearts, and I just don't get how you could go through your life knowing you left a sick child in the hospital."

Another nurse said she had a friend, a fellow nurse who, despite warnings not to get personally involved with the babies they cared for, adopted an abandoned baby. The infant had been so sick that she spent a very long time in the NICU, and during that time they became attached. "Sometimes these things sort of work out," she commented. "But I feel for that poor child, just knowing that her real mama could do such a thing."

The babies mostly slept, like little knit-capped and swaddled dolls; some of them wore foam goggles and rested atop jaundice-treating, bilirubin-promoting glow blankets. I'd see them flinch, their mouths moving involuntarily, their arms suddenly jerking up into the air. Sometimes the sudden movement set off an alarm. I persisted in thinking the alarms indicated heart failure or some other catastrophic problem, but the nurses kept assuring a hormonal, and easily rattled, me that it was common, what with such tiny wires and even tinier marks.

When it was time for me to leave—lactation served as a reliable reminder about Anna at home—I'd lay Lily back down in her isolette. She was so close, I'd think as I drove home, so nearly free of manufactured containers. From pipettes and glass dishes to catheters and incubators, she'd had so much assistance in her development and I was anxious for her normal, nonmedical life to begin.

Lily, apnea- and jaundice-free and breathing well on her own, came home on January 1, 2002, exactly two weeks after being born. As we gelled as a family, napping in the middle of the afternoon and waking up at dawn, Sophia helping to dress her sisters, snapping closed their special-ordered preemie nightgowns and pulling thimble-like socks onto their scrawny feet, holding their teensy hands in her relatively huge ones, I couldn't stop thinking about some of the women I had met in the NICU. A few always seemed to be there, having had severely premature multiples requiring aggressive neonatal intensive care, their babies inhabiting isolettes in a room I was not allowed in. The Filipino nurse from Lily's room, the one for the healthier or more fully developed babies, explained that the youngest and sickest babies needed an environment that mimicked a womb. The infants were fragile, she explained, their brains still developing and easily overloaded. So the lights were dimmed, and noises and activity were minimized. But I'd seen the parents in the family lounge and had been introduced to a couple of them by one of the neonatologists who cared for all of our babies.

"Man," I said to one new mom, as we surveyed the rows of suspended snacks in the vending machine; she had occupied a room down the hall from mine on the antenatal floor. "This is a lot of hospital time for you."

"You know?" she said, pushing a letter and a number and watching a packet of salted peanuts fall. "I didn't know how we were going to be able to afford having triplets. And then when I had to stay in the hospital for so many weeks I worried about that. But now that we're looking at God only knows how long in the NICU, I just have to stop thinking about it. Our insurance was already on thin ice, so I don't know what will happen. But as long as my sons are okay, I don't care about the rest of it."

According to Dr. Marc A. Fritz, chief of the Division of Reproductive Endocrinology and Infertility, Department of Obstetrics-Gynecology at the University of North Carolina at Chapel Hill School of Medicine, deliveries of high-order multifetal gestations in the United States have increased by nearly 400 percent for women in their thirties and by more than 1000 percent for women in their forties. An alarmed Dr. Fritz writes of the trend,

> Its causes are many and complicated . . . The technology itself is imperfect and carries intrinsic risk. Competitive forces and current measures of success encourage aggressive treatment by physicians. Anxiety, aging, and financial constraints imposed by an indifferent health insurance industry tempt patients and their physicians to pursue treatment and to accept risks they would otherwise avoid. The media, by celebrating high-order multiple births as a technologic triumph and largely ignoring the important underlying issues, distort the public's perspective and foster unrealistic expectations.

Dr. Louis Keith, president of the Center for the Study of Multiple Birth in Chicago, is a monozygotic, or identical, twin

and self-proclaimed "professional twin." He has studied twin-
ning for thirty years and worked with hundreds of scientists
who study multiples and thousands of mothers who have successfully or unsuccessfully dealt with multiple pregnancies. We
are currently experiencing, he believes, a national multifetal-
pregnancy and multiple-birth epidemic. Speaking of being in
the epidemic, smack dab in the middle of the exhaust-belching,
view-obscuring, DVD-in-the-backseat-playing epidemic, I notice it especially on the highways and byways, the school
pickup lines, and superstore parking lots filled with row after
gas-guzzling row of megavehicles necessary to haul around
one's bumper crop and its accoutrements. The car seats and
the strollers, the diaper megapacks and bulk cases of Hi-C,
adds up to a lot of stuff, a need for square footage, and a big environmental and social impact.

And as much as one praises the technology and lauds the
doctors (I do, I do), as much as one has profited by them and
enjoys driving her sports utility vehicle, the sheer number of
crowded simultaneous births brings with it a social burden.
The increase in risky obstetrical situations is driving liability
insurance for ob/gyns out of control. In some states, Texas and
Nevada being among the worst, women in their third trimesters
are scrambling to find replacement obstetricians as their old
doctors decamp in search of friendlier insurance venues. And
newborn nurseries have to devote often limited resources to
care for "iatrogenic multiples," Dr. Keith's term for ART-
induced high-order multiples.

Iatrogenic multiples are those that have been medically enabled, *iatros* meaning "physician" in Greek, and *genic* meaning "induced by." (For real-world examples, please see the
Feinerman twins.) The American Iatrogenic Association (AIA),
which is "devoted to the study and reporting of medical errors
that lead to disease and death," does not, however, mention assisted reproductive technology as among its concerns. The AIA
has examined optical chains making crummy glasses and ten

million women without cervixes still getting Pap smears and medical personnel skimping on hand-washing. But so far the AIA has not seen multifetal gestations as instances of medical error, harm, or ethical lapse. At least not yet.

Public schools must accommodate these children, some of whom have special needs as a result of their low birth-weights; their incomplete development and later cognitive delays place them at a higher risk for attention deficit disorder and other learning disabilities. School boards and parents of multiples are at loggerheads over who should ultimately determine class-room placements. Should traditional policies, whether they favor keeping multiples together or splitting them up when separate classrooms are available, be reconsidered? Should the decision always be up to the school (the rationale being that a school can serve as objective judge of a child's particular learn-ing style, while parents, especially ART parents, who feel that the sacrifices they made to have their children impel them to direct their every circumstance, lack objectivity to make good decisions for their children)? Or should parents, arguably the people who best know their own kids, have the final say?

I told Dr. Keith my own story, how I had three embryos transferred my first successful cycle and ended up with a sin-gleton, and three the second successful cycle and had twins, that I had a pretty bad time of it while pregnant with the twins, and that I was sitting on frozen embryos that I just couldn't get out of my head.

He interrupted me. "You got lucky. Leave well enough alone."

"I know. But I've just been giving these issues so much thought, you know, for the book and even before that. I've talked to the Archdiocese of Chicago and my rabbi and other people's rabbis and ethicists and theological students and friends and other people who've had to make decisions on what to do with frozen embryos. Really, I've sort of searched my soul, and I found no obvious conviction where frozen embryos are concerned, particularly since we can always donate them for scientific research, and frankly I feel like I owe science a big one. But don't I owe the embryos something? Isn't there a moral duty? An obligation? At the very least, I'd like to think I'm not the kind of person with a convenience default."

"The question is not whether one has an obligation to the frozen embryos," Dr. Keith said, clearly settled in his position, "but rather whether one has an even greater obligation toward oneself. By this I mean the maintenance of your health and the avoidance of the potentially catastrophic complications of multiple pregnancy that you dodged in your last pregnancy."

"I know it can be pretty rough," I said. "And I know how lucky we got. Me and the girls." *And Gary*, I meant to say but didn't. "But leaving well enough alone might have meant I never tried IVF in the first place, and then where would we all be?"

"It's a Pandora's box," he said. "Once you open the box of your next pregnancy, you have no control over what happens, and neither do your doctors."

The patient who sees a reproductive specialist does so to get pregnant, Dr. Keith explained. She visits the specialist's office, spends the hour or so that it takes for her procedure, easy peasy, and then goes home. But once pregnancy is achieved, the reproductive specialist's job is done, and a bunch of other people are left to deal with the results. First, the responsibility shifts to the obstetrician; once the woman delivers her babies, whether they are full term or far short of it, the obstetrician's duty ends. And so it is the parents, with arms and laps and sometimes incubators full of babies, who end up having to deal for a lifetime with their assisted reproduction. "With the increased rate of neurological handicaps and cerebral palsy that are associated with the high rate of preterm delivery and low birth-weight," Keith says, "the story continues for the lifetime of the children."

Dr. Keith explained that there is much about ART that no-body ever talks about, and that vast numbers of women so hate their experience with the first cycle that they never come back for more. I mumbled little assents. I respected his opinion and, more important, his work on behalf of multiples, and I appreciated that he deals with "catastrophic complications of multiple pregnancy" for a living and knows from whence he speaks. But still I wondered: wouldn't a woman forever regret leaving the Pandora's box alone when the truth was, she doubted it was a Pandora's box at all, just a plain old cryogenic straw containing embryos that might turn into kids as great as the others that, for one reason or another, hadn't ended up in the straw?

How could I leave the embryos frozen indefinitely when my timing largely accounted for the children I ended up with? If I had waited another couple of years to get started and Hamlin had been prevented, or strongly discouraged, from transferring more than one or two embryos, or if I'd met enough of the families struggling with triplets and quadruplets and been convinced to take it slowly, perhaps Sophia or Anna or Lily wouldn't have made the cut. Which, then, of my astonishing children might not exist? The sweet-as-sugar blonde, the funny and sensitive brunette, or the whip-smart redhead? Which of the Disney princesses—the Little Mermaid or Jasmine or Sleeping Beauty—wouldn't have a Feinerman girl representative?

From what I could tell, the cycles that worked seemed no different from those that failed; only the endings were spectacular in their differences. I had no magical feelings about the successful cycles, and no sense of doom about the failed ones. Each time through, whether the embryos were fresh or frozen, I made it my business to follow my doctor's orders (except for the preinjection alcoholic courage), neither skipping appointments or injections nor taking unnecessary risks. (Okay, L.A. hadn't been smart.) And as anxious as the early failures made me, as impatient as I was for a baby, and as hard as I swallowed each time I stuck my flesh with a needle, I never really hated

the IVF. Yes, I worried about health risks and dreaded the traffic and the hours in the waiting room and Carol's mood. But
I always considered myself vastly fortunate to have access to
such powerful medicine, such incredible science. I thanked
my lucky stars, and the generations of ancestors who met and
coupled when they had, for the coincidence of the technology
and my reproductive years. And I continue to thank my husband for being such a willing partner, and my girls for bearing
out my every instinct and decision.

11

Remain in Light

Outside Sophia's room is a storage closet filled with sealed plastic containers labeled neatly to remind me of their contents: "Girls, 6 to 18 months, PJs, leggings, tops." "Neutral, 2 to 3 years, sweaters, jeans, bibs." Through the milky plastic I can see the snap T-shirts we first dressed the babies in, drawstring nightgowns with flip-over mittens to keep them from scratching their own faces, yellow and lavender socks as thick as towels. There are summery dresses printed with butterflies, wee Levi's, and old rock concert T-shirts recycled into puff-sleeved blouses (David Bowie's feathered hairdo and catlike eye makeup adorably creepy on the backs of our toddling girls). The items are stacked between sheets of tissue paper, like a pastel timbale or a baklava.

In our basement is a room with a rust-streaked concrete floor, and the sound of dripping water that I've tried to trace to its source but cannot. Two strollers are parked in the corner — one for two babies, the other for one. There is a stroller base to snap a car seat into, two car seats, one bouncy seat, and a couple of high chairs. I go down there occasionally, to fix blown fuses, to stow and retrieve patio furniture, for bottles of wine, or to practice collapsing the high chairs and folding closed and popping back open the strollers. I try to preserve the girls' baby things, keep them functioning smoothly. I also like the memories they conjure. I look at the sun canopy on Sophia's old-fashioned pram, so ample it sheltered her not only from the sun and the rain but from my view as she tossed aside a store's worth of hats, toys, and snacks on our walks. The high chairs remind me of the foods the girls liked, pears and orzo and full-fat yogurt and their first birthdays with the ceremonial slabs of cake, the way they grabbed big handfuls of devil's food, squeezed it through their fingers, and watched as crumbs hit their bare legs and nestled into the seat crevices like a thousand little ants.

Like a newly thin person buying herself a bikini, I took seriously the selection of baby gear. It was my payoff, at least until I got to lay eyes on my kids, and I tried to choose items that balanced function and form, durability with some intangible quality, like a minivan's antithesis, to stoke my sense of myself as both mother and good ol' me. I thought little of expense and cared not how contemptibly yuppieish these elegantly engineered and supremely shock-absorbent conveyances were. I researched the different models, the various brands, double-checked items on parent review boards and *Consumer Reports*, and handed the final list over to my mother, stepmother, and mother-in-law, who purchased them as baby gifts. It was their way of helping us out, showering us with well-earned riches after our arduous reproductive ordeal. But more to the point, by being the ones to put these items beneath their granddaughters' darling tushies, the grandmas were involving themselves in the prosaic lives of these once-uncertain beings.

The girls grew fast, moving on to regular chairs and tricycles, leaving me to wonder whether this part of my life was finished, my body a repository for slowly failing systems rather than budding new ones. This apparatus, too, the tricked-out stuff that had once seemed so important, so crucial to get right lest I expose my children to harm, a recall, or Winnie the Pooh vignettes, over and done with. How long might it all remain down here, with me paying occasional visits with a dust rag or broom and envisioning not just the former occupants but other, future ones? I may never do anything decisive, may never go in for a frozen embryo transfer, wavering until I hit forty-five or so, then realize that the thought of having more babies at such a reproductively advanced age has become a joke, the punch line in a midlife crisis shtick, a pathetic and desperate attempt to continue seeing myself as fruitful.

And anyway, I'll tell myself, the kids and Gary and I are getting too old and set in our ways to change our domestic setup. And anyway, we need that corner for the more recently defunct things—the tricycles and wagons, the caved-in dollhouse. Until one day, on a Tuesday or Friday, garbage days on our block, I'll drag everything up the stairs and out to the curb, the massive metal frame of the pram scratching the wall as a constant reminder of what we'd given up, and I'll watch from the window as the garbage men toss it all into the back of their truck, rugged mountain-touring wheels spinning in the air as the truck rumbles down the street, a neighbor's Dell box wedged inside the high chair. But for now, while I'm not yet too old and we still have our frozen embryos, I work the levers and wipe off the dust to keep any rust from settling in.

The cryopreservation storage tanks are airtight and familiar-looking, like a five-gallon Gatorade dispenser meets a South American percussion instrument meets a submarine. Metal handles jut off to either side of a postcard-size blood-orange "biohazard" sticker, its three interlocking circles like a symbol for unity or a half-assed Olympics. The lid is hinged at the back and locks down in the front with casters on the bottom, allowing the tanks to be wheeled away and tucked out of sight.

Embryos to be preserved are sucked into straws—plastic or glass capillary tubes—with the patient's name, procedure date, and embryo classification information (number of cells and whether blastocyst-stage) indelibly printed on the outside. The straws are sealed before being frozen. The freezing process itself is controlled and completed in stages: the embryos move gradually from body temperature down to −196 degrees Celsius and are bathed in cryoprotectants to prevent cellular harm. The straws are placed inside tubes attached to aluminum canes and are then plunged into a liquid-nitrogen-filled storage tank called a dewar. At one cane per patient, and several patients per dewar, the number of dewars at cryobanks is ever increasing as more and more people go through ART and leave behind their perfectly good but unnecessary extras.

In a frozen embryo transfer (FET) cycle, Lupron is used to suspend a woman's natural hormones while estrogen and progesterone supplements are added to produce the ideal hormonal environment. Hormone levels and uterine thickness are checked by blood test and ultrasound, and when everything is synced up and primed, the embryos are thawed at room temperature over the course of about an hour. Once thawed, they're washed to get rid of every last trace of cryoprotectant and placed in embryo culture medium for resumed development in vitro.

At this stage the level and degree of cryodamage becomes apparent. If more than 50 percent of the cells remain viable, the embryo is considered to have survived and to be still capable of establishing a healthy pregnancy. At less than 50 percent, an embryo has partially survived but wouldn't be chosen for transfer. If all the cells die, the embryo is classified as "atretic." Around 65 to 70 percent of embryos survive thawing, 10 percent partially survive, and 20 to 25 percent are atretic. Data suggests that embryos with 100 percent cell survival are almost as good as never-frozen embryos, implantation rate–wise, but only about 30 percent of embryos endure that well.

The primary factors in predicting pregnancy rates from frozen embryos are the number of embryos transferred and the quality of surviving embryos, including the number of surviving cells and the embryonic morphology (cellular quality and degree of fragmentation). Some peculiar factors also affect survival rates. Embryos that were produced using ICSI survive in higher numbers, and those with an even number of cells (two, four, or eight) survive 5 to 10 percent more often than those with an odd number of cells, and embryos created from donor eggs have a 2 to 5 percent greater survival rate than those from infertile women.

Approximately 400,000 frozen embryos are stored in around four hundred fertility clinics around the United States. According to the CDC, frozen embryos were used in approximately 14 percent of all ART cycles in 2003. Diminished success rate aside (26 versus 34 percent), there is much to recommend a frozen cycle. It costs only around three thousand dollars for the various tests and drugs and procedures—way less expensive than full-on IVF. It's less invasive, and no stimulation drugs are involved, only the birth control pill and some Lupron to take medical control of a cycle, a week wearing an estrogen patch, some progesterone gel inserted where the sun don't shine, a few blood tests, and an ultrasound to see that the hormonal and uterine environment are ripe, and then the transfer and the bed rest and the waiting and the pregnancy test.

In 2003 the ASRM surveyed ART clinics to get a handle on their frozen embryos—how many there were and what people had slated them for. According to the respondents (340 practices out of the ASRM-registered 430 returned their surveys), nearly 88 percent of frozen embryos are targeted for patient

use. Of those stored in clinics for other reasons, less than 3 percent await donation to research. Slightly over 2 percent await
destruction per patient request, and another 2 percent await
donation to another patient. A tiny number, well under 1 percent, are being stored for quality-assurance checks. Still another
4 percent are there for "other reasons," including lost contact
with the patient; abandoned; patient death; awaiting a disposition decision; embryology training; wishes not specified on
permit/no permit; divorce case, awaiting final decision; and
awaiting transfer to long-term storage.

All of this technology—the mind-blowing possibility of freezing sperm or eggs or embryos for future use, and the permuta-
tions this possibility suggests—was sixty years in the making. In
1948 scientists attempting to freeze fowl sperm mislabeled a
couple of compounds, substituting glycerol for whatever freezing solution they intended to use. The glycerol made for a
thorough and quick freeze, and in 1972 preimplantation mammalian embryos were successfully cryopreserved, leading to a
new branch of science that, at its apex, includes the preserva-
tion of reproductive material with assisted reproduction patients, and animal breeders, its foremost beneficiaries.

In animal breeding, frozen stock assures that only the best
stuff gets passed along: out with the mangy and swaybacked, in
with the sleek and stallionesque. In the 1950s scientists began
successfully using artificial insemination to enhance the genetic stock of dairy cattle. Reproductive technology—artificial
insemination and embryo transfer alike—gave breeders a way
to intensify their use of nucleus, or elite, animals. By improv-
ing reproductive rates of the top animals, fewer were needed,
therefore restricting the range of genetic possibility, a good
thing when trying to produce cattle with squirtier udders or
beefier haunches. In the same way, reproductive technology
gives people (me) the chance to intensify their (my) use of su-

perior breeding stock; an elite, nucleus type such as Gary contributing half the DNA of our frozen supply, assuring me that our kids will have at least some shot not only at less beefy haunches but at being tall and enjoying gloriously thick hair and going to Stanford. It also gives women without a fertile male partner and men without a fertile female partner the chance to choose genetic characteristics as described on gamete (egg or sperm) donor bank menus.

Embryo transfer in animals was first performed in 1890, when Sir Walter Heape of the University of Cambridge transferred two Angora rabbit embryos into a gestating Belgian hare doe that he referred to as a "foster mother," resulting in a mixed litter of Belgians and Angoras. Embryo transfer in food animals began in the 1930s with sheep and goats and continued in the 1950s with pigs and cattle, the idea being that the reproductive potential of a genetically important animal can be realized only by increasing her output. The way to increase output is through embryo transfer, letting other, less genetically gifted but still uterus-endowed animals bear as much surplus offspring as possible. Freeze elite mama's embryos, ship them around the world, and watch the heads of cattle increase not just in number but in shapeliness, the sty sweetened with the porcine ideal.

In humans, the Australian doctors Alan Trounson and Linda Mohr produced the first successful IVF baby from frozen embryos in 1983. By 1988 sixty-seven American clinics had FET programs, and hundreds of babies, so-called "frosties," had been born. But as vociferous as the consumer demand for cryopreservation became, clinicians had their reservations. In the first place, they didn't want to be accused of engineering "designer babies," an accusation made more provable since embryos were in suspended animation, a perfect state for performing preimplantation diagnosis. Clinics also wanted to avoid the politics surrounding prenatal embryo adoption, abandoned embryos, and the disposal of unwanted embryos.

Some also forecasted an unnerving social future, with widows seeking to have their deceased husbands' babies months or even years after the tragic event, widowers showering new brides with a dead wife's eggs, and divorcing couples fighting over the embryos like any other custodial trophy.

There have been no demonstrable physical problems with pregnancies or children resulting from FET. And the domestic animal industry, which has frozen and transferred embryos on a large scale for decades, has seen no increase in birth defects. Still, experts worry about tampering with genetic development, particularly by such dramatic means as freezing and thawing. As Lord Robert Winston, Professor of Fertility Studies at Imperial College School of Medicine at London University, has said, "Basic functions such as growth, respiration and metabolism are regulated by genes. And if you change the way those genes are expressed—even temporarily—during times of rapid development, such as an embryo, you may well expect to see changes in the way the embryo develops." His laboratory at Hammersmith Hospital found that, indeed, freezing embryos impacted "the normal activity of vital genes." But as with other assisted reproductive technologies, which are all relatively novel, nobody knows the long-term implications, if any.

Some ethicists, including those on the President's Council on Bioethics, raise concerns over the social implications of freezing embryos and their constituent parts. They mention the possibility of posthumous parenthood: how a serviceman on the eve of shipping out to a battle zone might make a deposit at a sperm bank; the specter of his newly minted widow arranging to harvest her still-warm husband's sperm by way of assisted sperm retrieval. Such scenarios bother Leon Kass, who chaired the council from 2002 until 2005, provoking as they do his "yuck reaction," a litmus test for biotechnologies that Kass terms "the wisdom of repugnance." The council also ponders the potential damage not only to a resulting child, but to

social attitudes toward and understanding of family relationships, of "mother" and "father."

Blastocyst-stage embryos represent a significant potential
source of the embryonic stem cells that could be used to grow
replacement tissue for people suffering from a variety of diseases, like Alzheimer's, Parkinson's, cancer, and diabetes. Such
stem cells have the ability to grow into just about any cell in
the human body. But the President's Council, conservative
members of Congress, and scores of conservative groups worry
about using frozen embryos for scientific research; they find
it repugnant to even consider destroying potential human
life, no matter the promise for scientific advancement. They
showcase "frosties" as proof that these embryos are nascent
people—wheelchair-bound and tremor-stricken human beings be damned. Proponents of stem cell research argue that
tens of thousands of these embryos will be destroyed anyway
and that using them productively is an ethical solution. The
debate continues: in July 2006 President Bush vetoed a bill
that proposed the alternative-to-destruction solution. Meanwhile, science's ability to create embryonic stem cells has
sparked bitter debate not only on stem cell research but also on
embryo adoption, abortion rights, cloning, and the appropriateness of federal funding of human embryo research.

Ignoring, for the moment, romance and a shared sensibility,
dimples and gray-green eyes, and the fact of the Talking Heads'
Remain in Light on the tape deck when he picked me up for
our first date, my gut instinct that Gary was the man for me was
absolutely evolutionary. The height, that hair, those shoulders—it wasn't hard to zero in on him as the source of some
primo material, a genetically superior fellow. I'd dated my fair
share of potential mates. But between the pipsqueaks, the
pushy, and the ambitionless, the one with an ear trained on the
voices in his head and those that failed my yuck test, my reproductive yearnings weren't piqued until I met Gary, whose babies, as the story goes, I couldn't have without some help. So

we'd employed ART and ended up with an overproduction that, like an animal breeding program, gave us flexibility. But in a breeding program it doesn't much matter how many calves a cow has—there being no future college bills to consider, no summer activities or carpools to arrange, and no arguments between heifer and bull, as the bull tries to unwind and enjoy his *New Yorker*/baseball game/daughters/dinner/beer, about the light at the end of the demanding-babies tunnel. But having frozen stock has presented us with a major league dilemma.

We have three outstanding children who generate more joy than we ever could have imagined. They make friends easily, respect authority, and are generally healthy, Sophia's past health blips and Anna's frequent ear infections notwithstanding. They're typical children, sweet and naughty, dutiful and obstinate. There's no autism or ADHD, no Beckwith-Wiedemann, bladder exstrophy, or any other IVF-implicated problem. In short, there's nothing to warn me against having more IVF children, except my husband and parents, some friends, and the rational portion of my brain.

The girls are emotionally tight, close in age, and have had the benefit of parents in their thirties, if benefit that be. They're potty-trained and socialized, burgeoning readers and dynamite conversationalists. They're a pack, the three of them, and I should count my blessings, I am told. I shouldn't be greedy lest I open a can of worms to ruin our perfectly good lives. *But it's not a can of worms,* I think. *It's a vial of human embryos, our embryos, with the potential for human essence and a soul, the potential to be a baby and a kid, to learn how to swim and do fractions, to like certain songs and one political party or another, to come home from college at Thanksgiving and call us in the middle of the night with news of a towed car or a new baby and not, as one might think, as I once thought, mere blobs of undifferentiated cells.*

I have a friend who had four children the easy way, boom, boom, boom, boom, and is now hell bent on a fifth, despite a newfound difficulty in achieving and sustaining pregnancy. She's been to Hamlin's office and knows what to expect and the risk of multiples, but is raring to commence ART. I, by contrast, would be happy enough leaving well enough alone, if only I didn't have leftover embryos. I'd always pictured having three kids, just as my parents did. Three seemed like the right number to prevent people, namely us, from stacking one child up against the other. And while we are not a small family, three children are hardly unwieldy, a zone defense functioning just about as well as man-on-man.

Gary and I have honed our negotiation skills among the three. We've figured out how to discipline them, plan and organize social events, and enrich the things they learn at school. *You're right, Lily. You do know how to paint your fingernails with a permanent marker.* Adding another child to the gelled mix would be a gigantic leap of faith. But true as that is, we've already created, and saved, a handful of embryos whose destiny I feel compelled and duty bound to fulfill. And if bladder exstrophy or a rare retinal cancer waits in one of those dewars, so be it.

We had embryos frozen at two separate facilities, the five in a dewar up at Gamete Resources and an additional twosome at a facility called Reproductive Genetics (RG) that stores embryos for Hamlin's downtown practice. We assumed we'd used up our frozen embryos, thawing them all and transferring the best three, when we underwent our unsuccessful frozen embryo transfer. Turns out we hadn't—a snafu that was undoubtedly Hamlin's fault but that I couldn't be angry about, realizing that a different progression might not have yielded my present children. And anyway, how could I ever be angry at Hamlin for anything, really?

Our cryopreservation budget was seriously overspent. I sent payment to Gamete Resources: "Annual Storage Fee of Cryopreserved Embryos" was itemized in the "Description" portion of the invoice, "500.00" was listed in the "rate" section, and days later I also received a bill from RG. I ignored it, thinking it some sort of nonidentical duplicate, a fraternal invoice, until I got another bleeding "past due" stamp making plain there'd been no mistake. I called RG and left messages on their system voice mail. I called Gamete Resources. A guy in the lab named Manny confirmed that they had five but knew of no others.

When the double bills arrived the following year, I launched an aggressive phone campaign, leaving three and four messages at RG, one after the other, slowly spelling my name and clearly stating my Social Security and phone numbers. I also left word about my mounting anxiety and dismay. This was not only my property they were sitting on, I emphasized, this was my *biomedical* property, my potential *children*. A woman finally called, confirming they had a record of two blastocyst-stage embryos frozen in March 1999 under my name and "Social."

"Are you sure they're mine?" I asked.

"We haven't made a mistake yet," the woman said. "It'd be bad for business. So you want them, then? Or should we keep them here? Whatever you want."

I wasn't sure what to do, so I called Hamlin, who was surprised, thinking we had thawed that entire batch. He urged me to borrow one of Gamete Resources' transport tanks and fetch the two in the city. I'd want to have them all in one place for when we made our final decision, he explained.

"I think we want to go ahead and try a transfer," I said, not having finalized a decision with Gary, but more and more convinced that I couldn't live with any other. He said that'd be fine, that I should speak with the woman in his office who coordinated frozen transfers. He also mentioned that the old freezing methods lagged behind the 2001 technology, the vintage of our second batch.

"But the ones in the city are blastocyst-stage," I said.

"That's good, but truthfully, it probably won't make much difference. The attrition rate with those older embryos is considerable, even though they're genetically younger. Young enough, in fact, that if you did conceive using them, you wouldn't necessarily need amniocentesis! But like I said, we didn't really know how to freeze embryos without damaging them back then. Maybe there'll be a perfect one when we thaw them out. But if you're worried about a surplus, especially with this discovery of two more, you should keep in mind that we may only end up with one decent embryo."

Of course I worried about a surplus—purging our existing one was the reason I was even talking to Hamlin. But if we were to agree to FET, I'd have to figure out the most responsible yet morally acceptable way of handling the seven without creating additional problems. We could thaw them all out and choose the single best. But then, whether or not I ended up pregnant, what of the other embryos that had survived the thaw but hadn't been chosen? I'd still know they'd been discarded, their condition worse now than before we'd decided to do anything.

Thawing them out one by one presented other quandaries. If I got pregnant with the first, there'd still be six, and what then? Thaw out number two, put it in, and keep on going until there were none, a kind of Russian roulette with accruing babies like bullets to the head? But thawing them out one at a time could be enormously expensive, to the tune of $21,000 at the current rate, leaving me, after seven-plus months of estrogen patches and progesterone gel and negative pregnancy tests, a very unhappy mother of three. But I was loath to risk a multiple pregnancy, knowing how we had barely evaded tragedy the first time through and remembering Dr. Golden's warnings against future ones. And I knew myself better than to believe I could selectively reduce. My newfound fundamentalist leanings were the reason I was even agonizing over the embryos. So consider an abortion just to play things safe? Lord, no.

I already had the forms, for when we decided how to proceed: whether to go for an FET, dispose of the embryos, or donate them for research or rearing. RG's release was straight-forward, containing a couple of signature lines to show we'd read, understood, and agreed to their rules for transporting frozen embryos, that we'd employ an approved cryostorage tank for the move, and that we'd make haste getting to the waiting facility lest we damage or destroy the embryos.

For Gamete Resources, we were to complete a "Consent to Receipt and Disposition of Cryopreserved Embryos" form, the same one I signed when I was going through fresh cycles to clarify our intentions. We were asked to circle a number between one and five representing the number of years we wanted our embryos stored. We were asked to indicate what we wanted to do at the end of five years; the options included donating the embryos to an appropriate recipient, which would entail additional medical, genetic, and psychological testing, or discarding them.

The Gamete Resources form had on it an explanation of their position on cryopreservation and the ownership, control, and disposition of cryopreserved embryos based upon their best understanding and legal counsel. They clarified that it was subject to change depending on legal developments in Illinois or other jurisdictions. Their disclaimer stated:

> It is our policy that embryos produced by the joining of eggs and sperm are subject to the disposition in a manner mutually agreed upon by the couple receiving ART services at the site except in cases of divorce. In the event of the end of a marriage, the disposition of embryos from a donor cycle shall (1) be the decision of both parties if both donor eggs and donor sperm were used: or (2) if one of the partners produced gametes, then he/she shall have the sole decision-making authority. The partner who supplied the gametes has full authority over the disposition of the embryos . . .
>
> Except where applicable law requires otherwise, or where a court has acquired jurisdiction over the embryos,

any decision regarding the embryos shall be the joint decision of the partners receiving ART services and shall be con-
tingent upon their mutual consent or upon a legally binding
and enforceable agreement, in writing, signed by both of
them.

Following that were listed several options in case of divorce
or separation, including donation to an appropriate recipient
or disposal according to lab procedure. Other choices included
ceding all embryos to the female partner, who then would
have full authority over their disposition, or to the other partner
(other than female, presumably), who then would have authority over their disposition. In the case of sperm and egg donation, the signatories had to clarify that they understood that
these fully donated embryos fell within the purview of both
parties. However, in a case of biology being destiny where lab
decisions are concerned, if one of the partners produced his or
her own gametes, he or she would have sole decision-making
authority. In the event of death, mental incapacity, or disappearance, the nondead, nonincapacitated, and nondisappeared
signatory could request that any and all cryopreserved embryos
in storage either become the property of the surviving partner
or be discarded according to lab procedures.

The fact of frozen embryos, our ability to freeze and store
them indefinitely, and the ability of either a woman or a man
to make plans as to their disposition with or without involving
a partner or an ex, simply on the basis of a contractual agreement, have raised sticky legal issues. So far they echo the abortion debate, as questions swirl around not only the morality of
destroying unused embryos but also who makes the ultimate
decision. In addition, the technological component has fueled
the imaginations of prognosticators who envision a boundless
and morally unmoored future. They posit gestating men, human fetuses placed in the bellies of cows, man-made fetal
incubators, and they question how these eventualities might

affect the abortion debate. They see a future in which abortion is no longer a question of a woman's right to control her own body, because if the fetus is separated from the maternal body, no longer is gestation a matter of a woman's physical boundaries, no longer is it her right to decide what will or will not happen within those borders.

Once pregnancy is taken out of the equation, no longer does a mother have a clear, direct claim over a fertilized embryo, no longer can she argue any variation on squatter's rights. Once an embryo can exist outside the mother's body, in a nitrogen tank or anywhere else for that matter, no longer is pregnancy a condition shared by woman and embryo. The fact that frozen embryos occupy neutral territory, medical territory, makes the question over their disposition one for both biological parents.

In November 2005 *The New York Times* ran a piece about the difference between abortion and frozen embryos as they involve parental rights. In the 1991 abortion case *Planned Parenthood v. Casey*, wrote author Pam Belluck, the Supreme Court held that a woman does not have to notify her husband when she is seeking an abortion. Belluck posed a hypothetical in which a woman seeks to become pregnant with frozen embryos while her ex-husband opposes it. Whose decision is it? In abortion cases the law has generally sided with the woman, but thus far in cases involving frozen embryos, judges have given equal weight to the father's view. Some courts have said that even if a contract exists specifying that the woman has a right to the embryos in the event of divorce, that contract would be unenforceable. As June Carbone, law professor at the University of Santa Clara, explained of a 2000 Massachusetts court decision, "Either parent cannot be forced to become a parent in circumstances where they object, even if they signed a contract."

The use of frozen embryos, unlike abortions, does not involve a woman's "physical integrity," the term used by Carbone. And fathers' rights groups may end up using the embryo issue to gain leverage. In fact, a Chicago lawyer and fathers' rights advocate, Jeffery M. Leving, has created a print advertisement aimed at fathers in embryo battles. "Dads, protect the fate of your potential unborn children," it says, taking a page from the right-to-life style guide. In cases in which no resolution can be found, courts have almost unanimously ruled that the embryo cannot be implanted.

In 1992 the Tennessee Supreme Court heard a case involving the disposition of seven frozen embryos as part of a divorce settlement. The case began as a divorce action filed by the husband, Junior Davis, in which the parties agreed on every term of dissolution except for "custody" over the frozen embryos. Mary Sue Davis, the wife, asked for the embryos, intending to transfer them to her uterus after the divorce. Junior objected, stating he wasn't certain he wanted to become a father outside the bounds of marriage. The trial court determined that the embryos were "human beings" from the moment of fertilization and that Mary Sue, to whom they awarded custody, should be "permitted the opportunity to bring these children to term through implantation." The court of appeals reversed, citing Junior's constitutionally protected right not to beget a child where no pregnancy has taken place. The appeals court held that both parties "share an interest in the seven fertilized ova" and remanded the case back to the trial court.

Mary Sue, questioning the constitutionality of the appeals court's decision, brought the case to the Tennessee Supreme Court. On review, the Tennessee Supreme Court acknowledged the "obvious importance of the case in terms of the development of law regarding the new reproductive technologies." In the meantime both parties remarried, and Mary Sue changed her mind about the frozen embryos. She decided it would be best to donate them to a childless couple, a transaction that Junior opposed, preferring to discard them and be done with it.

Unlike Gary and I, who had to clarify our intent in case of incapacitation or divorce (reflexively, we ticked off the small box next to "donation to research"), the Davises hadn't executed a written agreement specifying disposition. Moreover, no Tennessee statute governed the use, storage, and disposition of frozen embryos, since most of the state laws that bear directly on the clinical practice of assisted reproduction are primarily concerned with questions over access. Over the past couple of decades, however, anticipating these sorts of embryo-ownership issues, some states have begun passing legislation.

A 1986 Louisiana statute forbids, among other things, the intentional destruction of a cryopreserved IVF embryo. It refers to embryos as "in vitro fertilized human ova," biological human beings, who are not to be considered property; be it of the physician who acted as the agent of fertilization, the facility employing him, or the sperm and/or ovum donors. In addition, as a juridical person, an in vitro fertilized human ovum cannot be owned by the IVF patients, who owe it "a high duty of care" and prudent administration, who must resolve disputes in its best interests, and who, in case they renounce their parental rights to it, must make it available to another couple for "adoptive implantation."

A 2000 South Dakota statute makes it a Class I misdemeanor to knowingly subject an embryo to any research that is "not intended to help preserve the life and health of the particular embryo subjected to risk." Governor Mike Rounds signed a 2004 bill that bans human cloning, stem cell research, and any procedure that places the nucleus of one cell into another. Although it was rejected by the electorate in November 2006, Governor Rounds also signed an abortion ban earlier that year, which he described as a direct challenge to *Roe v. Wade* and which was timed to take advantage of anticipated changes in the Supreme Court's makeup.

The ban is based upon the idea that "life begins at the time of conception." The language reflects this idea, using the term "unborn human being" to describe an individual living member of the species throughout the entire embryonic and fetal ages of the unborn child from fertilization to full gestation and childbirth. While the law doesn't explicitly address frozen embryos, the definitions undoubtedly apply and would likely be used to resolve any disputes over embryonic disposition. That is, until the law is deemed invalid for violating current constitutional doctrine. Or until South Dakota enacts specific pro–frozen embryo, anti–breathing person legislation.

Other countries are beginning to impose time limits on the storage of biomedical materials. In parts of Australia frozen embryos may be kept in storage for a maximum of five years, and eggs and sperm for ten years, after which time they must be removed and donated to another couple, used for training and quality assurance tests, or handed over for research, depending on the availability of a licensed project. One can also request an extension. Similarly, Gamete Resources uses five years as its upper limit; the term can be extended, but the regulation forces patients to reflect on their embryos each half decade. Because embryos can be kept frozen for an indefinite length of time (the birth of healthy babies from decade-old embryos has substantiated this bit of science fiction), people hold on to them, paying their yearly fees and reupping their five-year terms. But clinics also report vanished patients, invoices returned to sender, and sender forced to reckon with orphaned embryos.

According to the American Fertility Association (AFA), fertility doctors have concluded that the key to their patients' happiness is to make a decision, no matter what is ultimately decided. When people donate their embryos to research, they say, it lends them a sense of closure. Like a pagan bow man offering a hunk of meat to the God of Hunting, it's a way of giving something back to the outfit responsible for one's bounty. It also provides reassurance that one's efforts, one's embryos, will have some enduring value. Those who decide to discard their extras find relief in having gone full circle, in concluding unfinished business. It's not the idea of disposing of embryos that bothers these folks, but their very existence.

The doctors in the AFA survey didn't plumb the psychology of frozen embryo donors, perhaps because many donors are religious, and religiosity and psychology are hard to peel apart, or perhaps because of the extreme emotional complexity involved. The researchers did, however, acknowledge how logistically and emotionally complex donation can be. To that end, the ASRM has established guidelines requiring a six-month quarantine of the embryos, blood tests for the recipients, and blood and genetic testing of donors. Donors and recipients must also sign informed consent documents, in which the donors relinquish parental rights and the recipients accept them, should a child result. In addition, both parties are strongly urged to get psychological counseling.

According to the 2003 ASRM survey, only 2.3 percent of the estimated 400,000 frozen embryos in storage are designated for donation to other families. A Northwestern University study found that 30 percent of couples with frozen embryos initially say they'll donate extras to another family; then three years later, up to two-thirds of them decide against it. Faced with the reality of having to undergo counseling and STD tests, and the realization that the embryo they'd give away is their born child's full genetic sibling, they retreat.

I get this sentiment. Having nothing to do with a pragmatic concern about accidental incest (the rationale Orthodox rabbis give for disapproving frozen embryo donation to another couple), and everything to do with my kids representing the best of all possible endings for our embryos, I just can't imagine Gary and me not being the ones to try to fulfill this potential. As we ready the girls for bed, going through the bedtime paces and brushing and flossing and reading stories, we look out the window and each of us chooses three unique things: magnolias scattered on the gravel, a small white flag stuck into the lawn, the Dohenys' upstairs lights on across the street—and I can't help but think what a good group we are, how lucky another child would be to be a part of us, how lucky we'd be.

We have room enough for another, live near great public schools, know the various deadlines for AYSO registration, and have ongoing relationships with piano, gymnastics, ballet, and art teachers. I have a husband who participates fully and a babysitter whom the girls adore. We have the car seats and strollers, the boxes of clothes, and variously shaped breast-pump attachments. And I'm going to give away the raw material that might possibly turn into the infant who would ride in the seat, stroll in the pram, and drink all that expressed milk?

Donating embryos to research seems noble, but before I'd even consider it, I'd want some sort of assurance they'd be put to prodigious use. No skimming or waste, no United Way–style defrauding: I'd insist that 100 percent of 100 percent of the embryos be used productively. *Make like an Inuit*, I'd tell the lab guy before signing the papers, *and use every last bit of what you kill—the cellular equivalent of meat and bones, skin and fur.* In fact, I'd make a list, asking that one cell go toward cancer research, another for Parkinson's, one for juvenile diabetes, and another for IVF advancements and so on, until I was satisfied that my embryos and I had contributed not just to the greater good but to mankind's salvation.

The Nightlight Christian Adoptions agency founded the Snowflakes Embryo Adoption Program in 1997 to find homes (uterine and beyond) for frozen embryos. By that year, crappy freezing methods aside, substantial numbers of these unique and fragile "snowflakes" were accumulating in U.S. cryobanks, a situation that Ron Stoddart, executive director of the program and an adoption attorney, couldn't abide. He wanted the embryos to "realize their ultimate purpose—life—while sharing the hope of a child with an infertile couple."

Nightlight believes that life begins when an embryo is created and that embryos are preborn children waiting for a chance at life. Receiving families must be screened and counseled; the general profile thus far has been white Christian couples who agree not to abort any of the embryos they receive. An adoptive mother must be physically able to carry a pregnancy to term, and a letter from a doctor must confirm her fitness as a hedge against a medically indicated abortion. Applicants must state their commitment to providing the child with a "constructive, wholesome and spiritual home environment." The donating couple can also designate criteria for the recipient, specifying, say, a Christian family that includes a stay-at-home mom of a certain age. The goal, at least as stated in Nightlight's material, is to complete the "cycle of life and build loving families." Realizing this goal is helped, in large part, by a million-dollar federal grant administered by the Department of Health and Human Services to increase public awareness of embryo-adoption programs.

In June 2005, as reported in *The New York Times*, a conservative Christian Bellevue, Washington, couple with three children heard about the Snowflakes program and mobilized themselves to act on behalf of the "pre-born children." They believed the Lord was calling on them directly, telling them to try to give one of these children a shot at life. But they had their concerns: mostly the husband worried that paying money for the frozen embryos would fuel an evil, life-disregarding fertility industry. (While the embryos themselves are free, there are fees associated with their transport and with the medical procedures.) So he spoke with a Southern Baptist church elder, who assured him, "If you want to free the slaves, sometimes you have to deal with the slave trader."

The couple acquired thirteen embryos from an Austin, Texas, fertility clinic and ended up having a son. Along with twenty other abolitionist families, they attended a May 2005 White House event arranged to showcase embryo adoption as the ethical alternative to stem cell research. At the event President Bush declared that there is "no such thing as a spare embryo," and the parents proudly showed off their "snowflake" babies, kissing them and hugging them, pumping their little fists in the air and pointing to their pint-size "Former Embryo" and "This embryo was not discarded" T-shirts.

The term *embryo adoption*, rather than the AFA-preferred *embryo donation*, is an example of language creep, an attempt to linguistically equate, and onward into the eardrums and brains of the people who hear it, the status of embryos and children. Some frozen embryo advocates argue that embryos, frozen or not, are children at an early stage of development. As Ron Stoddart put it, "We have adopt-a-pet, adopt-a-highway. I personally feel that a child is going to feel a lot more comfortable knowing they were adopted as an embryo than knowing they were donated." Opponents of the term point out that *adoption* implies a specific legal framework that applies only to living children, and that in forty-nine of these fifty United States, "embryo adoption" isn't legally recognized; only Louisiana has passed a law proclaiming embryos to be "juridical persons" with full human rights.

An ASRM spokesman told *The New York Times* that proponents of embryo adoption "have an explicit political agenda to actually take away choices from infertility patients." Proving this point, Bill Saunders, director of the Family Research Council's Center for Human Life and Bioethics, maintained, "Our position on IVF would be you shouldn't create through IVF more embryos than are going to be implanted, and we don't think any should be frozen. But when it's clear that a couple is unable to or unwilling to implant an embryo—that basically they've abandoned the child—then we see embryo adoption as a solution to the problem."

Jean Bethke Elshtain, a political philosopher and professor at the University of Chicago Divinity School, thinks people should be required to make a determination about the fates of leftover embryos before undergoing a single ART procedure. More important, she believes that destruction, whether by research or disposal, should not be among the options. Pondering the constant creation of spare embryos, she worries that lacking options and storage space, society will have little choice but to disseminate them commercially, buying and selling them for research, or to dispose of them. Elshtain recommends we enact a system of restraints, both ethical and legal, that allows the science to blossom but that checks its potential side effects and abuses.

RG lists "embryo adoption" rather than "donation" among its offerings. Perhaps it's just a matter of semantics, a relaxed usage of a loaded term. Or maybe the person in charge of designations there believes that embryos are early humans stuck at a cellular stage. RG's "Embryo Adoption Wish List," a worksheet for would-be adoptive would-be parents, asks them to specify their preferred maternal and paternal characteristics, including ethnicity, religion, ancestry, eye and hair color, hair type, skin tone, freckles, height, build, and education. Gary and I didn't have to provide this information when we froze our embryos. If we were the ones to use them, who cares what potentials those tiny bundles contained? We'd want them no matter the Russian peasant stock. But if we decided on donation, we'd have to examine ourselves and describe our findings in a way to attract potential parents. I'd need to confess my tendency toward freckle clusters beneath my nose that resemble Hitler's mustache. I'd have to remember my real, unhighlighted hair color and come up with a descriptor that, unlike *mousy* or *dishwater*, doesn't conjure rabid pests or dirty sinks.

And then we'd have to wait, feeling insecure if our embryos were repeatedly passed over. We'd want to defend them, plead their worth to the overly picky donees who we'd have no choice but to assume were some kind of anti-Semites— otherwise who wouldn't want embryos whose parents had attended prestigious colleges and grad schools, a six-foot dad and a mother with a hair color described on the form as "winsome wheat"? I'd find myself turning into that Texas cheerleader mom, going to the mat for our progeny, even if it lacked hands for holding pom-poms or thighs up which the white boots could reach.

Clearly, Christian embryo-adoption organizations are not the only folks intent on humanizing frozen embryos. In infertility chat rooms and IVF blogs, the infertile and their readers refer to them as "embies," assigning nicknames having to do with their frozen state: Icy and Frosty, Crystal and Snow White. They post photos with descriptions like it's an annual Christmas letter. "Frosty is a perfect blastocyst who managed to survive the thaw and transfer! The embryologist had such nice things to say!!"

One blogger invites her readers to "meet" two of her newly received embies, darlings she hopes will now "snuggle in." Three images accompany this invitation. The first shows two embryos stagnant beyond mere photographic freeze, as if fossilized or made of cement. The second catches one of the embryos hatching, a small circle pushing beyond the larger round orb of the zona pellucida like a two-tiered snowman. The last image shows the embryos immediately upon introduction into the uterus, a speck inside a larger, shadowy space. The writer, like any boastful mother, compares them to twinkling stars.

Notes from other women, fellow IVF travelers, suggest the common view that embryos are children of a sort. They call each other "Mommy" and congratulate one another on their "beautiful babies." They mock-scold the children, telling them to heed their mother and "implant as told." They write effusively, as if gazing upon newborns, marveling at their teenytiny fingernails, their silky complexions and goosedown hair, rather than fuzzy photos of frozen cells that mainly resemble smudged contact lenses.

Is their notion of embryos as children a kind of shorthand or boiled-down discourse expressing profound reverence for human life and a deep appreciation for the passion of maternal yearnings? Or do these "mothers" truly believe in embryonic personhood? Do they consider each embryo an individual human being with a concomitant moral status? When they name and tease these earless, brainless cells, do they count down the weeks until they'll be rockable, burpable, diaper-soiling people, whether nudged along by science or left to fulfill an intrinsic intention? And if indeed they believe in an embryo's humanness, would they oppose research that would destroy it, even if the tests were aimed at upping their very own conception odds?

Not every conception begins a life; not every pregnancy results in a birth. Still, the Catholic Church says that an embryo must be treated "like a person," a developing human being who should be granted the full protection of an actual human being, neither to be used for research nor destroyed. In Jewish law, frozen embryos may be used by the contributing couple for future pregnancies or passively destroyed. That is, an embryo may be allowed to thaw out and die on its own, but nothing can be done to hasten its demise. Orthodox rabbis object to embryonic research since it is an active process resulting, ultimately, in embryonic destruction. They also object to donating embryos to other infertile couples, since the risk that genetic siblings will meet and marry outweighs any perceived benefit.

Leon Kass, who uses the idea of "natural law" to frame his approach to bioethics, maintains that certain natural goals must be respected, and that every organism, human life in particular, ought to be created only through natural processes. In 2003 the President's Council issued an overview of IVF technology that referred to an embryo as "nascent human life," "nascent life in vitro," and "child-to-be," worrying moderates and reproductive rights groups alike. This overview, an early version of the final report, suggested that every embryo created in the United States should be tracked and records kept of its outcome, and that a federal registry of IVF children should be created. In this initial report Kass fiercely opposed IVF, but the final report was muted, embryo-as-young-baby-wise, and suggested only mild regulations rather than enforced Orwellian registries. It also acknowledged the difficulty of regulating the ART industry, particularly for a conservative administration, pitting as it does libertarian market values against religious ones.

In its final 2004 report, *Reproduction and Responsibility*, the President's Council acknowledged that embryo research has the potential to benefit both infertile couples and people with diseases or disabilities that could be cured, or at least ameliorated, by regenerative medicine derived from embryonic stem cells. But the fact that the research requires the use and destruction of human embryos caused the council to assess it as ethically untenable. As it stated in the report, "To regard developing human life as a mere means—even a means to a noble end, such as the alleviation of suffering—presents a moral problem with potentially serious consequences for society as a whole."

The report enumerates the potential social problems, including a coarsening of sensibilities in the general culture and conditioning respect for life on a life's possessing certain capacities. The council also dismisses the ethical validity of creating embryos expressly for research, again since it would tend to simultaneously devalue and commodify human life, and coarsen cultural sensibilities. The conclusions reminded me about my own ethical misgivings over my carnivorousness and how I steadied them by pointing to the fact the meat had been farm-raised, existing explicitly for its marinade bath, time on the grill, and rendezvous *avec* my taste buds.

Although Kass was originally opposed to IVF, he now says he sees no harm in it for married couples, particularly since time has proven its relative safety, both for the women who undergo it and for their IVF-enabled children. "Nobody knew in advance that in vitro fertilization would be, by and large, safe,"

Kass says. "It's not that I think the activity is absolutely innocent [in moral terms], but on balance, one could justify its use for infertile couples. And having known some such children myself, one is simply delighted they are here." Amen.

I once knew where I stood on most moral issues. While I'd never pull the wings off a butterfly in exchange for a hefty payout, I'd yank with gusto if it'd save a human, or even a canine, life. I've never stolen anything or lied on a timesheet, never justified underpayment by claiming that a rich corporation doesn't really need my money, you're welcome Starbucks, and word up, there's an Evanston barista trying to foist free shots of espresso and pastries upon a certain upright citizen who truly only wants what she orders, freebies from The Man, the pilfered Kenyan and covert scones striking her as too poisoned to accept. I was firm in my modern humanism, rejecting supernaturalism and relying on reason and science, democracy and compassion. And my exposure to the miracle of ART, both in the lab and in my children, has only strengthened my devotion to science and my steadfast belief in looking after human needs in the here and now. (I refer to a democratization of essential human fulfillment, rather than a Kobe beef in every pot or a Hummer in every garage.)

But, even while my veneration of science has been strengthened, resulting in an almost unspeakable appreciation for the ability of human beings to extend human life, to cure disease, and to cure infertility, I have a new respect for the ability of cells to develop into more complex beings—into, well, children. I also fully realize (and am trying to integrate into a broader philosophical understanding) the ways in which my present circumstances, our seven frozen embryos, have forced upon me a moral flexibility; my beliefs have swerved a lot farther to the right than I ever thought possible.

I have a newfound reverence for all human life, whether gestating or just plain existing. I also want those brilliant scientists to keep up their research and do what they can to improve our lot, health, and life spans. And if it's embryos, more and more embryos, that they need to succeed, I'll strive to secure them—lobbying and fund-raising and calling on IVF clinics myself. Only, hands off ours—they're taken, earmarked for possible future personhood. And as these ethical questions continue to arise, I'll keep on exploring my new moral elasticity to see where its limits lie. It'll give me something to chew on, whether I'm in the hospital on bed rest, or simply enjoying a juicy burger, farm-raised or not.

12

We Are,
All of Us,
Bears

On May 29, 1968, in the middle of the night, my mother's water broke. Having already been through it once before, she anticipated the pain to come, the moment, just as her baby crowned, when a nurse would plaster an anesthesia mask over her mouth, the fact that she'd not be awake to greet her newly born newborn. I arrived at six a.m. on May 30, weighing six pounds, thirteen ounces, and measuring nineteen inches. I had a thick shock of hair that my mom pinpointed, once she regained consciousness, as the source of her unrelenting third-trimester heartburn, and swollen lips that helped me take the bottles offered in lieu of my mother's breast. We stayed at the hospital for five days, normal back then, and on June 4, the day before Robert Kennedy's assassination, an event my mother claims to have foreseen during the final days of her pregnancy, I came home.

Mine was a typical late-1960s birth, my conception a similarly standard affair, there being only one route back in the day. And even as I try mightily, nay excruciatingly, to repress thoughts of my folks in conception mode, I can somewhat imagine what went down. Certainly there's a backstory—my parents having gone out of an evening, perhaps, taking in *Oliver!* or *Funny Girl.* Returning home, my clean-cut dad would have fixed himself a scotch, my Mary Tyler Moore look-alike mother putting on a satiny smocked nightgown, tuning the radio to Otis Redding or Marvin Gaye, pulling back the quilted bedspread, and reading Anaïs Nin while her husband finished his drink.

A lot has changed since my parents' encounter almost forty years ago (although Marvin Gaye's ability to lubricate the wheels of romance endures). In that time their relationship soured, and they divorced, leaving my brothers and me to marvel that they'd ever been a couple, that we'd been conceived at all. But more to the point, kids nowadays need not assume they resulted from parental sex. My brothers and I, on the other hand, were forced to listen to Jimmy Mercado, a school bully with a cruel streak made even more brutal by his ability to turn his eyelids inside out, eyelids that presumably didn't blink while he, as he claimed, spied on our parents through their bedroom window, catching our father in the act of "screwing the shit out of our mother." Thinking that he'd seen my dad wrenching actual BM from my mother's body, I was horrified, never mind the intended image. Schoolyard taunts about copulating parents carry a blunted wallop now that a child's mere presence no longer serves as smoking gun.

On the flip side, children can now doubt their biological relationship to a parent or sibling. And as potentially willies-generating are thoughts of one's parents making like a workbench, alternate conception scenarios may be even harder for a child to digest, especially those that feature biological relationships outside a family's prosaic ones or that involve contentious custodial struggles. Whether or not a child's particular conception narrative includes donors or surrogates, finding out

that one was conceived in a relatively new way can be destabi-
lizing. Of course, ART is increasingly common, downright
ubiquitous in some parts. But children like to feel they're no
different from their parents or peers, and for those conceived ex
vivo and in vitro, there's no denying that their initial earthly situation diverged spectacularly from the customary one.

Along with sleeplessness and worry, illness and online stalk-
ers, daughters who beg to dress like skanks and little assholes
like Jimmy Mercado, one of parenthood's biggest challenges is
explaining difficult concepts, especially those that still baffle
us. Even harder is volunteering ideas we know will forever alter our child's consciousness, particularly when we remember
the way our own parents bungled it. My mom told us that a
good friend of hers—a second mother to us—slept with other
people's husbands. My dad mentioned that a friend of his, a
great guy, the life of the party, was a *schicker* and a cheat. He
told us about the atomic bomb, the ability of one country to
wipe out another with the push of a button; my mom told
us that Vietnamese people eat dogs, most people hate Jews,
women who get abortions eventually lose their minds, and that
my dad emotionally suffocated her, all of these tidbits etching
themselves indelibly in my mind.

Certainly some people handle knotty topics well, effective
communicators who triumph at metaphor, folks who are just
completely in tune with what and how and when their children need to get information. The clumsier among us do our
best, relying largely on intuition and, when that fails, on props.
Society has handed us assorted crutches for when the going,
and the curiosity, get tough. There's organized religion, ani-
mism, and spiritualism. There's also Disney with its history of
animated animal deaths, Bambi's and Nemo's hapless mothers, and Simba's father, his luminous, astral spirit reminding
his son, and our children, not only that there is a circle of
life which includes its termination, but that death be not
tone-deaf.

Joining the ranks of hairy concept and potentially shocking account is ART. Discovering that one was conceived in an unconventional way, or that his mother is neither a biological relative nor the woman who birthed him, can be a toughie, even if the child belongs to a community that supports IVF. Some experts think it is neither necessary nor healthy to share with a child the circumstances surrounding an IVF birth. They worry that societal opposition puts these children at risk of emotional damage, that what matters is the child's birth itself, not how it was achieved. No harm, no foul, in the form of revelatory heart-to-heart.

Adoption rights advocates, among others, disagree. They say that all children have a right to know where they come from, whether it be an orphanage or a fertility lab. In cases in which donors or surrogates participated, they argue, the children have biological relationships beyond their parents and a right to full disclosure, even at young ages and definitely before adolescence, lest revelations affect a teen's struggles around identity. Many parents who conceive by egg donation fear that they'll unwittingly be given somebody else's genetic material, and unknowingly rear a child who isn't a genetic relative, but studies show that more than half of such parents do not share the fact of egg donation with the children that result.

Since genetic inheritance is central to one's health, I'd argue that a child should get the pertinent facts at some point. I've also watched enough daytime TV to recognize that revealing a big family secret like "I Ain't Your Daddy" or "She Ain't Your Real Ma" often does not end well, either for the chair-throwing, TV-censor-triggering, boot-camp-and-detox-facility-requiring child, or for her beleaguered parents. Admittedly, that's not how it always goes; plenty of families weather intimate revelation more healthily and, at the very least, less publicly.

Clinical psychologists tend to agree that sharing information about reproductive beginnings with a child is healthy, but only if done in an appropriate way that takes into account their emotional and cognitive capacities. When preschool-age kids wonder whence babies, simple explanations can be offered. As a child advances, asking the inevitable, pointed questions, parents can unfold the story bit by bit, adding details as appropriate, both biological and clinical. All ART narratives should include a few elements, however. First, a child should know that ART-enabled babies are born just like any other. They're the same as other kids, even if conceived differently. Second, parents should present a united front, letting their children know that they made the decision together and were equally delighted with the result. Finally, in cases where donors or surrogates participated, the children should know, simply, that donors or surrogates are generous people who help others become parents.

Answering the call for child-friendly information, and filling an ever-widening marketing niche, are X, Y, and Me books. Their alternative-conception series, *Before You Were Born . . . Our Wish for a Baby*, includes some impressively specific subtopics, with stories of an IVF Baby, a Frozen Embryo, Donor Insemination, a Donor Egg, Donor Sperm, a Gestational Carrier, Surrogacy, Donor Embryo, a Baby Conceived for Female Partners, a Baby Conceived for Male Partners, Single Mom—Donor Insemination, Single Mom—IVF Using Donor Sperm, Single Mom—Embryo Donation (Adoption), Single Mom—Donor Sperm/Donor Egg, Single Dad—Traditional Surrogate, and Single Dad—Donor Egg/Gestational Carrier. It's a list that'd make Pat Robertson convulse. But X, Y, and Me's approach, the gentle text and familiar woodland characters, goes a long way toward dulling the critical thunder, the charges that ART not only is an abomination against nature but also destroys traditional family structure by encouraging single and same-sex parenthood and by sacrificing the life, and afterlife, of the children who result to satisfy selfish parental desire. The sweetness of the books, their loving messages for ART-enabled families, demonstrates how very human is the impulse behind assisted reproduction and how thoughtful are the responses to these new sorts of families and novel sets of emotional concerns.

X, Y, and Me believes that parents have a moral and ethical obligation to disclose the alternative methods involved in their child's conception, and the earlier, the better. They recommend that parents be proactive, controlling when and how information is disseminated, not only to prevent a third party from spilling the beans, but also to guard against a child stumbling upon it and impairing his trust. Proponents of early introduction say that knowing his genetic history and parental circumstances can help shape a child's sense of self, rather than becoming the thing that sends a formerly self-assured and secure kid into a tailspin if he finds out the hard way that having two biological dads takes some technological finessing or that "Aunt Joanne" is actually his "genetic mother."

The books are well done, featuring rosy-cheeked Mama and Papa Bears and an all-American, jeans-wearing cub, an Iowa pennant slanted on his bedroom wall. They explain the elements of technological conception in a straightforward way, introducing terms like "lab dish" and "a special cell from a nice lady called a donor" as if discussing Goldilocks and her bowl of temperate porridge. The characters are wholesome and appealing, the Papa Bear resembling Ward Cleaver rather than David Crosby. There are no mad scientist types drooling over steamy beakers, neither animated winking sperm drilling into eggs nor psychedelic embryos splitting their cellular selves in dishes. Only the parent bears on a tandem bicycle headed toward a building plucked straight off the University of Virginia campus, all symmetry and pediments and blue jays fluttering here and there, a picnic basket bungeed to the back of the bike for some post–in vitro eats *sur l'herbe*.

Expressing the simultaneous longing and prudence of people who enlist technological means to have a child, Papa Bear tells his cub that "before we could see you, before we could touch you, we knew that we loved you." Papa Bear says, "The first time we held you in our arms, we knew our dream had come true." He describes counting his son's ten fingers and toes and admiring his cute button nose, reassuring the IVF child, and her parents, that despite the alternative conception, these are normal kids. The books are neither overtly religious nor unrelentingly scientific. They're geared toward families with complicated histories and toward children with unique beginnings. Through their use of stock characters from book to book, they also manage to convey a sense that all parents are the same, somehow. Whether gay or straight, single or part of a couple, biologically related or not, young or old, we are united in our desire to do right by our children, no matter the specific natal path. We are, all of us, bears.

Whether or not I order *Before You Were Born . . . Our Wish for an IVF Baby* to get this conversation rolling, Gary and I have it relatively easy, as far as IVF narratives go. We have no strangers to introduce our kids to, no "uncles" or "aunts" who aren't, really. Their mother and father are their biological kin. If Sophia, Anna, and Lily want to blame someone for their greasy skin or bad hair or impatience or bowlegs, they will need look no further than the toads in their own kitchen.

But that doesn't mean we won't face challenges, not only the usual pickle of explaining human reproduction and our sexual bodies, but also how best to describe where babies come from in a way that touches on the standard "dadas have sperm and mommies have eggs," and the alternate and more pertinent "doctors have medicine and mommies have a high threshold for pain." It'll be a soft sell, no blow-by-blow accounts of procedures or disappointments, nothing so technical and scientific as to make them consider themselves exotic, alien, or Frankensteinian. Our goal, besides making them feel secure, will be to elicit an appreciation for how much we wanted them, how important scientific progress is to the human condition, and how beautiful and not-to-be-taken-for-granted is daily life.

So, yes. At some point, when the girls ask us questions that require real answers and not simple mechanical explanations, we'll discuss reproduction and assisted reproduction. But until then, until they lead us into the conversation, I'll maintain my silence. Creation and IVF are heady topics, and I don't want to confuse my kids before they even know the basics or give them information they have no way of processing. But I also don't want my reticence to signal I take any of it for granted, that it's no big deal. I think ART is the biggest deal in the world, its increasing ubiquity proving, rather than diluting, how truly awesome it is, each additional baby born as a result its own universe of miracle.

I do, however, wonder what impact the ability to initiate fertilization artificially will have on my kids' generation: will it affect their perspective on motherhood and human reproduction, their attitudes toward romance and faith? Just as they already take for granted various domestic technologies that completely blow my mind, TiVo and high-speed Internet connections and four-hundred-compact-disc carousels and fax machines, which still impress the hell out of me. But I don't want them ever to stop appreciating either the science that enhances all our lives or the mysteries providing the interest.

As we go about our days, operating assorted gadgets and profiting by technological advancement, I trill like Mork newly landed: "Isn't that cool how we can watch one show and tape another and stop live TV and fast-forward through commercials? And look how thin my computer is! When I was your age, only people on TV had computers, and they were so huge they filled entire rooms. And we didn't have CD players. We had turntables and records that'd scratch if your cat jumped on them. And if you were allergic to cats, there weren't any shots to counteract it. And nobody had phones or DVD players in their cars." The girls look at me as if to say, "Let go of the past, Mommy." But I don't want to let it go. The past reminds me to be thankful, particularly since, in the old days, besides the warped albums and missed programs and Wite-Out and communal computer labs and cat-induced hives, there wasn't much a woman could do about her infertility.

I walk around the house noting the technology. From the refrigerators and vacuum packaging in the kitchen to the array of analgesics and antihistamines in my medicine cabinet, our domestic lives have been improved in so many ways. We have less drudgery and more freed-up hours to fill with soulful pursuits (or not). We live longer, suffer fewer bouts of salmonella poisoning and muscular ache, die less frequently in childbirth, and bear fewer stillborn babies. But we also have the risk that this science-enabled bounty could be used against women, particularly in places where we're marginalized. If men can decode female rhythms, if they can deconstruct our menstrual cycles and manipulate our pregnancies, certainly a woman's social position is imperiled in cultures that view women as man's instrument.

The once uniquely female capability to bring forth life, this awesome power that has sustained male awe for millennia, the subject of mythology and poetry, song and social structure, has been tampered with to the point of being disabled. If a woman's social position is already tenuous, what's to become of her when scientific know-how neutralizes her maternal force field? Taken to an extreme, but increasingly possible, if women are no longer even necessary for procreation, if male embryos could just be plucked out of the embryonic mix and allowed to gestate in an artificial uterine environment, why bother keeping around more than a whorehouse's worth?

———

Over the past decade or so economists and social scientists have tracked the impact of technology on consumer culture and human interaction. Bioethicists are beginning to focus on the ways alternative reproduction might influence a child's sense of self and his relationship to the world. One concern is that children conceived in alternative ways will lack the bi-parental origins that have always existed, the altered biological relationships among donors, surrogates, parents, and offspring confounding basic human relationships. And certainly we hear stories that fuel the concern, like the one about genetic siblings born just a few months apart. Their biological mother hadn't been able to maintain a pregnancy, miscarrying numerous times. So she asked her sister to serve as gestational surrogate, a role her generous sister gladly took on. Four months into the surrogate pregnancy, the biological mother, the original sister, discovered that she, too, was pregnant. There are tales of anonymous donors seeking relationships with their progeny, and vice versa, sometimes for the best and other times not. Sadly, there are custody cases involving biological parents who, through contractual loopholes and despite their best intentions, end up not being able to maintain a relationship.

In 2004 a California appellate court decided that an egg donor had no parental rights to her twin daughters, even though she contributed genetic material and helped raise those daughters. The situation involved a lesbian couple who dreamed up a plan to create a family in a way that'd involve both partners physically, one woman providing the eggs and the other carrying the pregnancy. The relationship ended when the women fought over whether the twins should learn they were biologically related to both of their mothers. The court held that the donor parent relinquished her parental rights when she signed an egg-donation consent form.

Justice Mark Simons of the First District Court of Appeals wrote, "What is legally relevant is the finding by trial court that the parties' understanding showed that they intended [one partner] to be the one to bring about the birth of a child to raise as her own." But having been presented with determinations to make and documents to sign pre–fertility treatment, I understand that our signatures may not necessarily reflect our true wishes. We don't think we'll actually ever be faced with a situation in which we'll need to dispose of genetic material or cede custody. We just choose whatever option approximates a best-case scenario, knowing somehow that Option A or B or C will never come to pass. *Our eggs and sperm and embryos will become children, and we'll be mothers and fathers to them. Now get this form out of here.*

As Jill Hersh, the lawyer for the donor, commented, "This woman had her children ripped away from her and has been made invisible. She's naturally more than disappointed and feels her children were let down by the legal system. There is no question in her mind that she is one of their mothers and nothing can change that." As for the children, their history will include memories of a mother who no longer has a legal right to them and who lives in a state other than the one their "mother" decided to move them to. And whether or not it would have been damaging for them to learn the truth of their biological connection to this now-absent mother, their permanent separation from this woman who loved them and whom they loved in return most definitely hurts.

Shannon Minter, legal director of the National Center for Lesbian Rights, called the ruling discouraging and the decision that the girls have only one parent an insult to the "ovum" mother. The center filed an amicus curiae brief arguing that assisted-reproduction laws should apply equally to both partners. "It wouldn't be any less devastating if the court ruled that twins couldn't see their father," Minter said. "It's cruel and causes a level of psychological harm that will haunt them the rest of their lives. And what if something happens to their birth mother . . . they are orphans."

The lawyer from the winning side, Diana Richmond of

Sideman & Bancroft, said the ruling "preserves freedom of choice for same-sex partners. Any other decision would have created messier laws that wouldn't have done anyone good in the long run." She said that the children's prior connection to their nonbirth but gamete-donating mother does not mean she should have joint custody. "Many people form relationships with parental figures who live in their household, but that doesn't give them the same status as a parent," she said. "What contact exists after a relationship is over is up to the legal parent."

Still, whether or not ART impacts definitions of "mother" and "father," whether it confuses a child over relationships with his parents or individuals outside his nuclear family, I have to believe existence, the fact one has a confusable brain and a breakable heart, is worth the strife. Life can be messy, but it has always had that tendency. There have always been single mothers and children being raised by people other than their biological progenitors. There have always been custody battles and fighting parents and children who weather them. It's not ideal, these muddled surrounds, but it is life. As long as one provides a child with a compelling and life-affirming narrative, as long as that child is loved and taken care of, is made to feel secure and part of a family, whatever that family looks like, he'll have just as good a shot at happiness and success as the rest of us imperfectly reared human beings.

As for me, my biggest concern is not that telling our three children about their alternative beginnings will cause them to consider themselves abnormal. It's that it'll trigger existential angst, challenging the idea that life has some larger purpose. After all, traditional conception entails a sort of beautiful mystery, the exact sequence and timing of biological occurrences shrouded within the body. It allows us to imagine we were inevitable, a single sperm, the one with your name on it, tearing like a Tomahawk missile toward the egg fated to comprise the rest of us. Once medication and technicians are involved, artificially promoting fertility and choosing gametes, wielding the various tools and producing, in large part, the end result, faith is necessarily tested and anxiety fueled.

Granted, ultrasound images of oneself at the cellular stage are pretty cool things to have, a real crowd-pleaser at the wedding rehearsal dinner or bat mitzvah slide show, just the sort of thing I'd put on my album cover if I had a band. But if life is so traceable, if one can know the motility rating of the sperm that ended up fertilizing the eighteen-millimeter egg that ended up being you, perhaps that'll have some impact, whether flattening one's perspective or creating a false notion that life is certain and tangible, its creation a matter of combining certain elements, its end a similarly discernible disassembling, all the moments in between a mere matter of shifting scientific formulae.

Maybe I'm wrong. Maybe man's scientific ability stems from a divine source, the hand of God leading the technician's, and all of the results sanctified thereby. In fact, maybe my daughters, these three blessed and soulful beings, bear out rather than disprove God's presence in artificially stimulated conception. Maybe the mere fact of their existence, their emergence in spite of the human interference, the potential obstacles at every step, the rusty speculae and sticky syringes, the clumsy technique and imperfect judgment, is proof that fallible man is no match for the Almighty Lord.

Meanwhile bioethicists are keeping a keen eye on the social impact of using technology to achieve once-natural processes. Just as experts blame technology, in part, for compressing experience and flattening out communication, bioethicists fear that human procreation will start to resemble public manufacture more than personal affair. For the most part, they are not concerned with more traditional modes of ART, fairly commonplace procedures like IUI or even IVF. What really concerns them is ongoing experiments whose repercussions could move human reproduction into dangerous, dehumanizing territory.

Of course, progress is a great and wonderful thing, and if not for scientific invention, my life would be so different as to be unrecognizable. From obstetrical care to early childhood inoculations to fluoride treatments to omega-fat-enriched eggs on down the line to IVF, I appreciate and profit from scientific progress every day. But in the category of just because we can do certain things, should we, come the following examples of continuing studies with vast social implications.

Scientists are experimenting with nuclear transfer, which involves transplanting the nucleus from a fertilized egg into an enucleated fertilized egg. It's like somatic cell nuclear transfer (human cloning), except that the nuclei derive from other fertilized eggs rather than from a somatic cell of a living person. Theoretically a resulting child could carry genetic material from three or four people: the male and female progenitors of the original fertilized egg and the mitochondrial DNA from the donor of the egg receiving the new nucleus. In 2003 Chinese scientists reported achieving a triplet pregnancy with such embryos, although none of the fetuses survived to birth, a result attributed to substandard obstetrical care rather than genetic problems.

Researchers are also investigating whether ovarian tissue from aborted second- and third-trimester fetuses may be developed in the lab to provide mature eggs suitable for IVF. In July 2003 researchers said they'd obtained ovarian follicles from aborted fetuses between twenty-two and thirty-three weeks gestation, which they were then able to culture to a secondary stage. The researchers are now working to improve the culture media to prolong the culture period, allowing the follicles to develop sufficiently to become a source for human eggs.

Although speculative, there is ongoing research aimed at engineering uterine-lining tissue ex vivo to give scientists insights into implantation. In fact, researchers have transferred human embryos to an artificial endometrium, where the embryos attached and began developing. The researchers ended the experiment after six days of sustained development, fueling speculation about the possibility of continued embryonic growth in uterinelike substitutes. Investigations are also under way into uterus transplants, to enable women with damaged or missing uteri to bear children, and into implanting human embryos into specially prepared nonhuman, mammalian uteri to study their development. So far there are no noteworthy results, only the fact of the experiments themselves yielding amazement and trepidation.

Some thinkers, Jean Bethke Elshtain among them, consider these sorts of studies, as well as some current ART practices, to be "socio-biological experiments." She worries about the impact on the children and acknowledges that human cloning may be only a few steps down this scientific road. "Can or should we ethically go forward," Elshtain wonders, "embark on vast and reckless socio-biological experiments, in the absence of decent knowledge of what will happen to the children?" Commenting that most IVF takes place in the context of a marriage, and therefore that the child's "emotional and ethical surround" is both "substantive and decent," she says that what concerns her is the emergence of children, depending on the ongoing research, in "truly bizarre ways." How, she wonders, will parents craft for these children a compelling story of natality that promotes a belief in their uniqueness and merit? If a child knows he developed in a petri dish or an incubator or a faux human uterus, if he learns that his father was a serial sperm donor or his mother an anonymous egg donor with no interest in the resulting child, what impact will this have on his sense of self-worth?

Biblical creation narratives actually help explain away some of these concerns. They make it clear that human beings are good only for the flesh and blood part of their children; it is God who endows the meaningful, the stuff that brings us to life. The Talmud states,

> There are three partners in man: the Holy One, blessed be He, his father, and his mother. The father supplies the semen of the white substance out of which are formed the child's bones, sinews, nails, the brain in his head, and the white in his eye; the mother supplies the semen of the red substance out of which is formed his skin, flesh, hair, blood, and the black of his eye; and the Holy One, blessed be He, gives him the spirit and the breath, beauty of features, eyesight, the power of hearing and the ability to speak and to walk, understanding and discernment. When his time to depart from the world approaches the Holy One, blessed be He, takes away his share and leaves the shares of his father and his mother with them.

In the Bible, God creates man on the sixth day, saying, "Let us make man in our image, according to our likeness." He fashions man out of clay and, even more important, gives man the capacity to approximate godliness through spirit, enabling him to develop the mind and character of God. The Bible, then, shows us not only that God was the numero uno assisted-reproduction pioneer but also that man's corporeal being doesn't much matter. Yes, our bodies are fashioned in God's likeness and are therefore not a complete waste of time. But the nonclay internal workings, the spirit and character and soul, that, no matter how one develops, whether poofed into being by God or painstakingly manipulated by a doctor, are what truly animate a person. We are composed of both flesh and spirit, earth and heaven, the lump of clay that forms our bodies a big pile of nothing until God bequeaths spirit.

For all of us struggling with religion versus science and miracle versus technique, this idea provides a remedy of sorts.

When we initiate conception using man-made technologies, we aren't playing at God's job, since no amount of scientific brilliance will give us the capacity to create a soul in vitro. There can be no spirit donor, no such thing as a soulologist. All man can do is scientifically simulate conception and let the miraculous, invisible part happen beyond the reach of magnification and ultrasound.

"God blessed them. God said to them, 'Be fruitful, multiply, fill the earth, and subdue it. Have dominion over the fish of the sea, over the birds of the sky, and over every living thing that moves on the earth.'" According to the Bible, God put people in charge of our surroundings, granting us permission not only to rule our fellow creatures but also to subdue the earth, bringing it into control, lessening its chaotic intensity. One can then argue that scientific progress, in its ability to combat disorder and disease, is therefore not only not heretical but sanctified.

"God saw everything that he had made, and behold, it was very good. There was evening and there was morning, a sixth day."

13

Urbs in Horto

The Chicago Botanic Garden, 383 verdant acres of paths winding through formal plantings, bucolic waterways, and naturalistic arrangements, was until the late 1960s swampy, combustible marshland. Certainly there were Chicagoans who braved the conditions, camping or fishing or ice skating on the ponds, an escape from their workaday urban lives. But as uninhabited as the landscape was, as much of a diversion as it offered, the mosquitoes were a terrific annoyance, the bog fires an unpredictable hazard, the lagoons a fetid cesspit, and the ever-present mud impassable for the average mid-twentieth-century citizen's non-four-wheel-drive ride.

In 1965, 128 years after Chicago's incorporation and its adoption of the motto *Urbs in Horto*, or City in a Garden, the Cook County Forest Preserve and the Chicago Horticultural Society agreed to establish and maintain a botanical garden in Greater Chicago. The only available land was on Cook County's outskirts, but it was well over three hundred acres, justifying the distance from city center. They broke ground that fall, and for the next three years solid, John Ormsbee Simonds, a pioneering modernist landscape architect, designed and implemented land masses, drainage systems, waterways, islands, and roads.

Unlike most botanical gardens and arboretums, which are developed from private, cultivated estates, the Chicago Botanic Garden was an entirely man-made reclamation of lowland marshes and polluted lagoons. In *The City and the Garden*, Suzanne Carter Meldman describes the colossal effort required to transform environmental wasteland into botanical idyll. "John O. Simonds tells of the three-year effort . . . to move earth and divert water for a whole new landscape of hills, lakes and islands from the scrabble and ooze of depleted fields and grossly polluted waterways. It was a formidable project, and at least one person's automobile was almost lost in the mud." But in the spring of 1972 the Chicago Botanic Garden officially opened to a vista-loving public.

Amid the garden's diverse specimens, its ten thousand discrete plants representing twelve hundred taxa of herbaceous perennials, vines, shrubs, and small trees, its relatively bug-free environs awash in the sounds of spraying fountains and docent-guided tours, Gary, Sophia, Anna, Lily, and I attended an event put on by Great Lakes Fertility. In the summer of 2005 we received a shiny, grass-green card urging us to CELEBRATE LIFE! on its front, a card I nearly threw away, mistaking it for an off-course National Right to Life solicitation. Curious as to how I had made it onto the pro-life mailing list despite my ongoing support of NPR, environmental defense, and Senator Joe Lieberman, I opened the card.

As it turned out, our IVF clinic was "proudly hosting" a party, a "family reunion" to "celebrate life and miracles," a "festive gathering of our patients and their miracle children!" We wanted to go. Not only did the invitation beckon—a monarch butterfly, rows of sunflowers, and stands of orange lilies hinting at well-planned merriment amid panoramic surroundings—but there'd be food, entertainment, and fun for all. Besides, we hadn't seen Dr. Hamlin in ages, not since moving to the suburbs, and we thought it'd be great to check in, that he'd enjoy seeing the girls. And we were curious about the party itself, who would come and what sort of program there'd be. We joked that it'd be a theme party with petri-dish penny tosses, Pin the Sperm on the Ovum, and giant, furry gamete mascots, the photo-op of our girls in an embryo's embrace. Like class reunions that feature one's yearbook picture on the name tag, a voluminous hairdo or prairie blouse giving away an earlier incarnation, perhaps our children would wear name tags featuring grainy pictures of them at the cellular stage.

Or maybe the party would be completely understated, its real nature concealed to protect the more sensitive among us, the use of the word *life* a deliberate cover, like a plain brown wrapper. I scanned the invitation for hints there'd be a condition for entrance, a focus group or a survey, a mandatory tour of my uterus before we'd be allowed to hit the buffet. But I found nothing irregular, just a lovely invitation to attend a sincere celebration.

I called the RSVP number and confirmed that, yes, they could expect us five Feinermans, looking forward to it, thanks for the invite. Gloria, the woman in charge of fielding responses, said, "No, we should really be thanking you. There'd be no party without our patients. Nothing to celebrate, and no one to celebrate with."

"How nice," I said. "We'll see you there."

We pull into the parking lot, inching along to avoid the throngs of toddling children and baby-toting adults. Car doors open all over the place, and parents stick their chino'd legs from backseats as they lean in to unbuckle their children. Amid popped hatchbacks and opened trunks and parent after parent pulling out strollers and diaper bags and wagons, we all make our eventual way toward the garden's main building.

As we walk past some bike racks, a couple of older men sitting on a bench ask what is going on—is there a twins convention or something? I explain it is a party for a fertility clinic.

"I figured it had to be something like that," one of them says to the other. "I knew this wasn't normal—so many of them. Fertility clinic . . ."

We keep walking. I am relieved that our twins don't really look like twins, but I don't like the idea of our kids being so casually discounted.

"It does seem kind of weird," I say to Gary, quietly so our kids and the other families won't overhear. "You know, when you see so many in one place." He is carrying Lily, tickling her so that she squirms in his arms, telling him to stop, stop, and then when he does stop, saying, again, again. Anna and Sophia are walking with me, practicing their skipping and tugging at my arms. "I wonder how many sets there'll be, how many sets in his practice. I'm sure Hamlin keeps track. Think they'd tell me?"

"It's none of our business," Gary says. "And anyway, who cares? We should just enjoy ourselves as a family. Participate in the activities, eat some good food, notice what's interesting, of course, but in a people-watching way and not in a strange-IVF-situations way. You know, not get hung up on any bigger pictures or details that aren't our concern."

"I just think it's interesting, all of these variations on family. But I can't help but worry what other people think . . ."

"Who? Those old guys on the bench? Screw 'em. They're dinosaurs."

"No, not them specifically. People generally. I hate to think people consider infertility treatments abnormal. And if they do, then what? Will they belittle our children or consider them any less valuable just because we had to juice their beginnings? And all that talk of an epidemic of multiples is, if you ask me, prejudiced. IVFist. You know, a cloaked bias against it or the people who undergo it or the doctors who perform it. As if we choose to have fertility issues! As if having children this way makes them less pure and us, their parents, less worthy or capable. Like the children equivalent of a mail-order bride. And yeah, there are a lot of twins these days, but so what? It's not like they're an automatic drain on the system. And I mean, look around. Do you think any of these parents of multiples consider their children symptomatic of an epidemic? Do you think they'd say there's any sort of problem at all? We underwent IVF willingly, we were presented with choices along the way, and we made our own decisions. So if an increased incidence of multiple births is IVF's worst side effect, I'd say that's some benign practice."

"You're assuming that everyone who has triplets wants them. You're assuming that people who end up with premature or sick twins can afford to take care of them. You're also assuming that serious problems dissipate once the children grow up, but as you know, sometimes there's a long-term impact. Really, don't write off other people's problems."

"You shouldn't write off their joy. Parenthood, especially the kind you work hard for, this intentional sort that we're a part of and that is the reason for this party, is a privilege. We're all so lucky. Not to mention, and I know it's not ultimately important, but"—I raise my voice, so that the girls can hear me—"how cute are our kids? How much do you want to eat them up?" I pretend to gobble up Anna and Sophia's hands, making chomping noises and causing them to laugh, as I knew it would, as it always does.

"Shhh," Gary says, chomping at Lily's shoulder, "it's immodest."

Bunches of balloons, green and orange and yellow, are tied to easels holding propped CELEBRATE LIFE! directional signs, arrows pointing straight ahead. We cross over a bridge, spraying fountains off to our right, swans gliding noiselessly, majestically, obliviously all around. A trellis drips wisteria over our heads, and Sophia and Anna scoop shed flowers from the ground.

We stand in the A–F row at a check-in table, familiar members of the Great Lakes staff working the sheets, scanning for names. There are a thousand people here, easily.

We get to the front of our line. "Feinerman," I tell the woman. "Oh, you're Gloria," I say, reading her HELLO, MY NAME IS sticker. "This is so nice of you guys to do. What a great idea. What a beautiful party. Was there any particular reason for holding it now?"

"Unofficially, it's to mark the birth of the one-millionth IVF baby born worldwide, which happened earlier this summer. But really, it's just something the doctors have been talking about doing for a long time, and we figured our numbers were perfect right now. You know, enough families to make it superfestive, but not so many that it'd be completely chaotic and impersonal. Anyway, I hope you'll have a great time. Your kids are adorable. Enjoy."

We walk in. There are Technicolor Care Bears—Love-a-lot, and Harmony and Wish, according to a thrilled Sophia, who grabs her sisters and tears off in their mobbed, matted furred direction. We look around. The huge tent is filled with families, young and old, extended and small. There are Latinos and African Americans, Indians, and lots and lots of white people. There are long buffet tables and metal ice cream carts, popcorn and snow cone and cotton candy machines. And everywhere you look, there are costumed mascots, with children clustered around them; parents and grandparents snapping pictures as their children hug the foamy legs hard enough to dent them, giving silenced high-fives, staring into the characters' mesh-screened eyes. In the middle of the tent there is a dais and a podium with a CELEBRATE LIFE! sign stuck to the front. Dr. Hamlin stands next to the stage, and a long line of eager families wait to pay their respects.

"Let's grab the kids and say hi to Dr. Hamlin," Gary says, "before they get too into the activities."

We wait—the kids are distracted by Strawberry Shortcake, who danced with them, nodding her giant bonneted head when they ask her, repeatedly, if she is the *real* Strawberry Shortcake. When we get to the front of the line, Dr. Hamlin gives me a kiss. "Liz. How've you been? I haven't seen you in a long time. You finished having babies?"

"We moved to the suburbs last summer and quit the health club. Not sure about more kids yet—I'm still working on Gary. So how are you?"

"Just great. How are you? Look at these girls. They're beautiful. Simply beautiful. Everything's good?"

"Great," Gary says. "Thanks for inviting us. This party is outstanding."

"Our pleasure. It's a pretty big group, no?"

"Huge. You should be so proud," I say.

"You have no idea. It's so gratifying. Nice to see you. Don't be strangers, okay?"

"Okay. Thanks, Dr. Hamlin. Thanks for everything."

"My absolute pleasure. Enjoy it."

We grab some lunch and, not finding any empty tables, decide to sit on the grass outside the tent, next to a pond. Ducks float around on it, a mother and five ducklings, small, brown, and still fuzzy. They skirt the shore, chasing after thrown popcorn, all of them, mother and babies alike, dipping their heads beneath the water for submerged pieces.

"Mommy?" Sophia asks. "How old are the babies? Five, like me?"

"No, they're younger," I say. "See how they're fuzzy instead of smooth and feathered? I'd guess they're only about a month or so."

"What's a month?" Anna asks.

"About four weeks," I tell her.

"What's a week?" Lily asks.

"Seven days."

"You mean like MondayTuesdayWednesdayThursdayFriday SaturdaySunday?" Sophia says.

In that moment I feel exactly like a parent, teaching my children the basics and appreciating them for forcing on me a thoughtful consideration of the world I can take for granted. We are a family of ducks, taking in what comes our way and looking beneath the surface.

A microphone squeals, and then a woman, the head nurse Carol, announces there will be a few short remarks. We have a decent view of the podium and a clear shot of the speakers' profiles, so we decide to stay put on the grass. Dr. Hamlin, two of his partners, and Debbie the embryologist speak, each welcoming us and thanking us for having faith in them to help us realize our dreams and for sharing our children with them at the day's celebration. They announce that the party will continue for a couple more hours and tell us to have a great time.

A deejay starts playing music on the lawn, not far from where we sit. Several of the mascots are over there, doing Ring Around the Rosie with children and each other. Our kids want to join them. The deejay, a young, urban hip-hop-looking guy, surveys the dance floor: a couple of toddlers bounce off beat atop chubby legs, a little boy gets swung back and forth like a pendulum by his two moms, and groups of older kids tap the mascots on their backs and run away. Gary, the girls, and I dance for a while, Gary showing them how to raise the roof, his palms turned up toward the sky, while I teach a disco dance I still remember from sixth grade. When the girls run off to follow the older children, promising me they won't tease any of the characters or topple the babies, I find a bench nestled in some flowering bushes at the lawn's edge.

I can smell flowers and grass and hear the low-pitched hum of bees behind me. The deejay, clearly briefed on his audience, plays song after song about enjoying life and family. The songs are generic, the sorts I've heard a thousand times—"We

Are Family" and "What a Wonderful World" and "Celebration"—but it is the first time my kids have ever heard them, and they are having a ball. They dart in and out of the dancing crowd, Anna following Lily following Sophia as they hug one favorite character after the next, Care Bears and the Cat in the Hat, Scooby-Doo, their dada, and me.

We receive a goody bag on the way out. In it are kid-size plastic sunglasses, tiny plastic frogs, clapping hands on a stick, lollipops, and bubble wands. There are stickers of Piglet and a children's photographer's card telling us to visit her website to view moments captured from Celebrate Life! 2005. There is also a flyer with a photo of the six members of the embryology team in their blue scrubs and cloth booties. They are in the lab, gathered in a group, two sitting, four standing. There's a microscope behind them, a computer monitor, and a Plexiglas stand holding erect a few test tubes. This is the lab where my eggs and Gary's sperm were maneuvered, the equipment used to initiate and monitor our embryos' development, the very place the girls, my family, began. This is also the place where the embryos that didn't make it stopped growing, the place where our seven frozen embryos remain.

I look at the picture and wonder whether these folks enjoy their work, whether they realize how profoundly meaningful it is and how thankful the beneficiaries are. I decide that, when we get home, we'll write a thank-you note, our children doing a drawing, perhaps. Maybe they'll draw the Care Bears, maybe it'll be the ducks. Or maybe it'll be their family, all five of us waving or holding hands or standing with one another. Our family.

ACKNOWLEDGMENTS

My immense gratitude to Sarah Crichton for understanding deep, impractical desire and for gambling on me. Thank you to my agent, Katharine Cluverius, who sought the best for this project and became a trusted advisor and confidante. To Rose Lichter-Marck, thank you for juggling so gracefully and for your creative contribution. To the experts (rabbis, priests, doctors, philosophers, bioethicists, and sociologists, to name a few) who answered my questions and offered some of their own. To Joanne Koidin for the many phone hours spent reading and laughing with crying newborns in the background, and Jennifer Arra for your thoughtful input about the book and the issues that still haven't been put to rest. To Susie Kramer for reading it through medical eyes, to Birdie Hancock who went through these things with me, and to Laura Lappin and Liza Zito for caring enough to wince at the material. To my many friends for sharing your experiences, for your openness, and for permitting me to put it in print. To Edyta Samulak for all your care and the gift of time to get my work done. To the doctors and their staff who fulfilled my dreams. To my professors at the School of the Art Institute of Chicago: Rosellen Brown, Sara Levine, Carol Anshaw, and Janet Desaulniers for urging me to write when it was hard and to lay off when it got too hard. To my family, who never stopped supporting me, and to my father, Allen Kohl, for relaying his pride, and to all of you for letting me tell our stories. In particular, to Robert Kohl and Abby Kohl for going above and beyond, for sharing office space and opinions and for making plain your love. My deepest gratitude to my mother, Barbara Kohl-Spiro. Without you, there'd not only be no me, there'd be no creative me. I value your spirit and am eternally grateful for your understanding. To Jim McManus, my greatest teacher, mentor and champion, hero and friend. Finally, thank you to my husband, Gary, not only for the keen editing and sense of humor about our travails and their broadcast, but for your tenderness and thoughtful approach to all you do.